DATE DUE

NOV 1 2 2011	

MEDIEVAL AND RENAISSANCE FASHION

90 Full-Color Plates

Raphaël Jacquemin

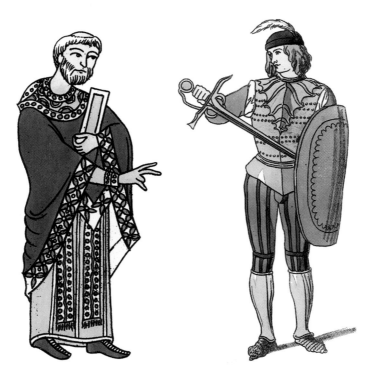

DOVER PUBLICATIONS, INC.
Mineola, New York

Bibliographical Note

This Dover edition, published in 2007, is a selection of plates from *Iconographie Générale et Méthodique, du Costume du IV au XIX Siècle,* published by L'Auteur, Paris, 1863 to 1868.

Library of Congress Cataloging-in-Publication Data

Jacquemin, Raphaël, 1821-1881?
    [Iconographie générale et méthodique du costume du IVe au XIXe siè-cle. English. Selections]
    Medieval and Renaissance fashions : 90 full-color plates / Raphaël Jacquemin.
        p. cm.
    "A new selection of plates from Iconographie générale et méthodique du costume du IVe au XIXe siècle, published by L'Auteur, Paris, 1863 to 1868"—T.p. verso.
    ISBN10: 0-486-45776-1 (pbk.)
    ISBN13: 978-0-486-45776-5
    1. Clothing and dress—Europe—Pictorial works. 2. Clothing and dress—Europe—History—To 1500. 3. Civilization, Medieval—Pictorial works. 4. Renaissance—Pictorial works. I. Title.

GT513.J2 2007
391.0094—dc22

          2006103548

Manufactured in the United States of America
Dover Publications, Inc., 31 East 2nd Street, Mineola, N.Y. 11501

List of Plates

16th Century

58. Flemish Noblewoman
59. Lombard Soldier
60. French Knight
61. Venetian Nobles
62. Nobility of France and Italy
63. Men-at-Arms
64. Flemish Squires
65. Flemish Noblewomen
66. German Nobility
67. Duke and Duchess of Bavaria
68. Pope Paul III
69. King François I
70. Noblewoman of Venice
71. Ferdinand, Archduke of Austria
72. French and Spanish Infantry
73. King Henry II
74. Princesses of Bavaria
75. Swiss Guard
76. German Foot Soldier
77. Coligny Brothers
78. Ladies of France and Germany
79. Italian Princess
80. Italian Ladies
81. King Henry III
82. Swiss Color Bearer

17th Century

83. Charles Emmanuel of Savoy
84. André, Cardinal of Austria
85. Pikeman and Harquebusiers
86. Elisabeth, Palatine of the Rhine
87. Jean Le Grott, of Lucerne
88. Halberdiers
89. Anne of Austria, Queen of France
90. Albert of Wallenstein

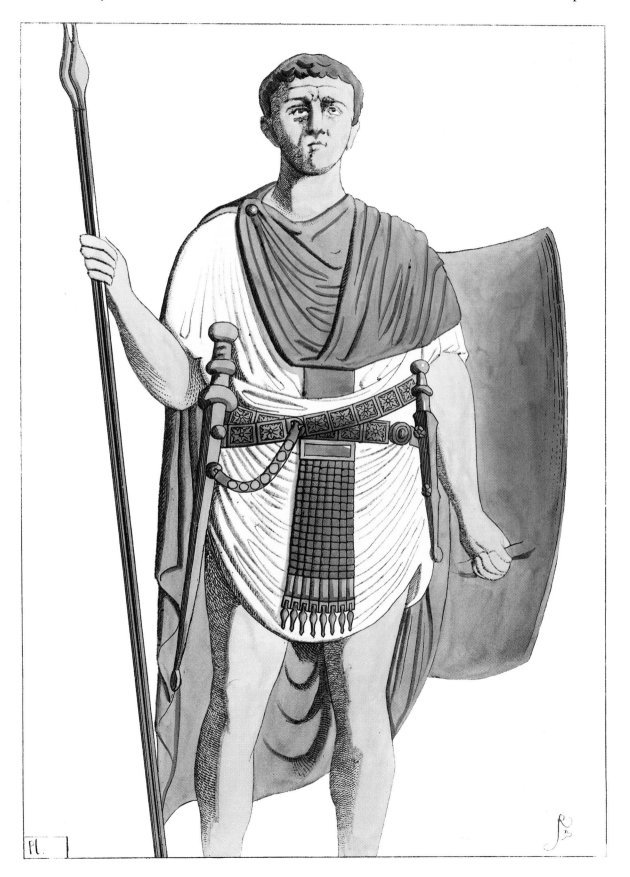

PLATE 1. Soldier of the 4th Dalmatian Cohort

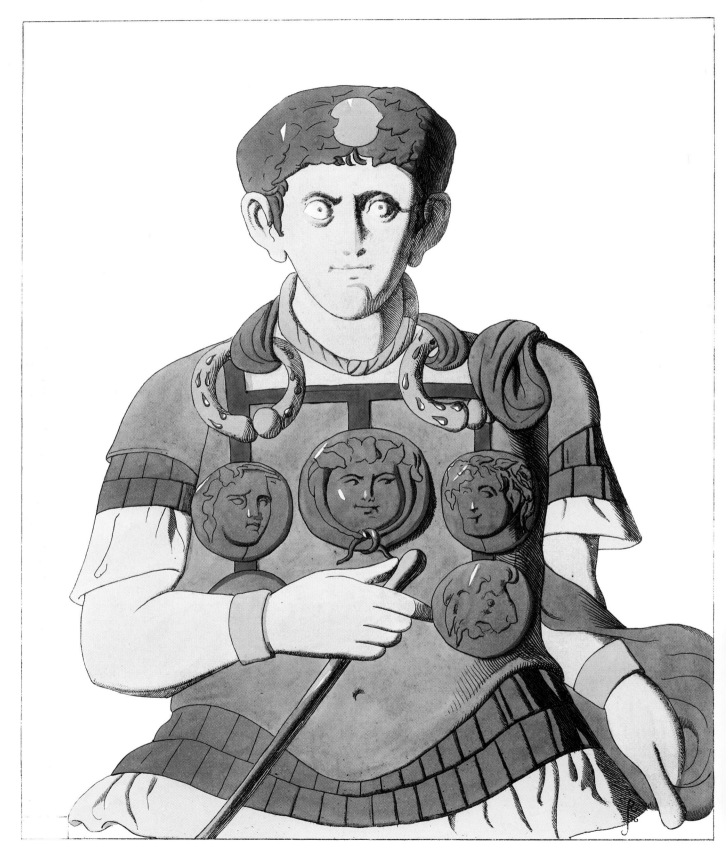

PLATE 2. M. Cœlius Lembonius, Legionary Centurion

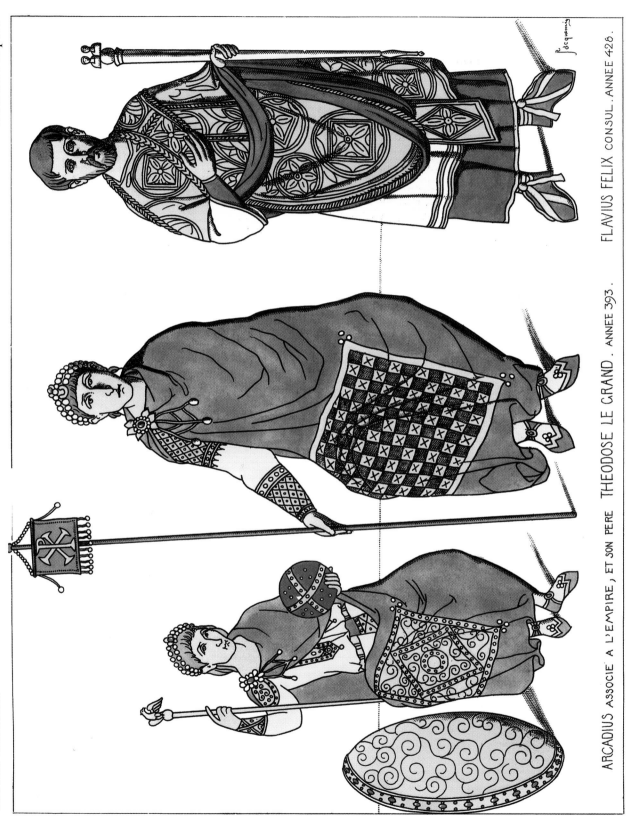

ARCADIUS ASSOCIE A L'EMPIRE, ET SON PERE THÉODOSE LE GRAND. ANNÉE 393. FLAVIUS FELIX CONSUL. ANNÉE 428.

PLATE 3. Arcadius, Associate of the Empire, and his father, Theodosius the Great, in the year 393.
Flavius Felix, Consul, 428.

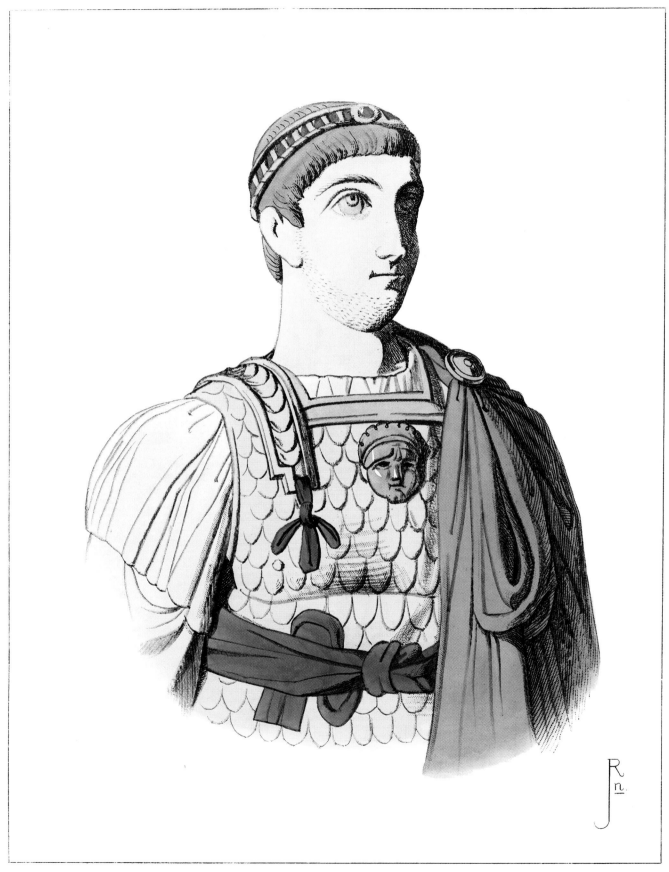

PLATE 4. Emperor Honorius (420)

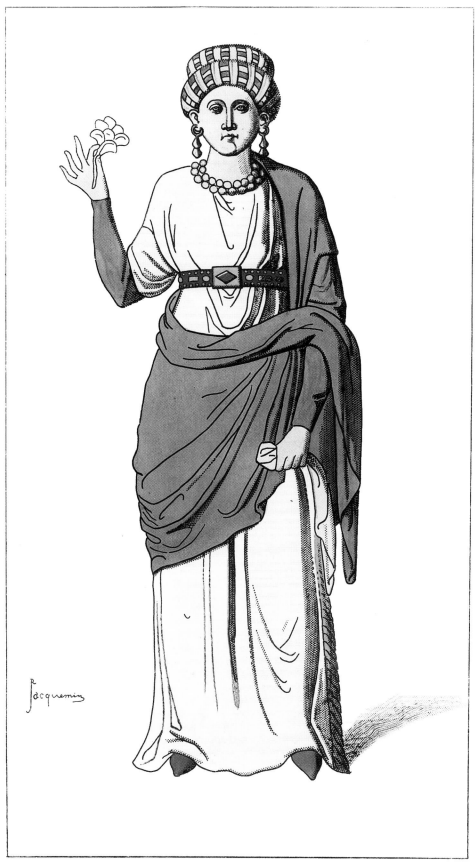

PLATE 5. Galla Placidia, Empress, Regent of the West, in 430.

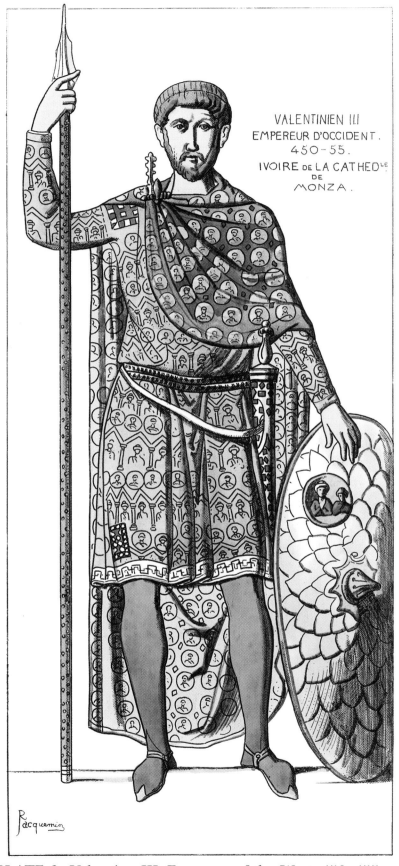

VALENTINIEN III
EMPEREUR D'OCCIDENT.
450-55.
IVOIRE DE LA CATHED^LE
DE
MONZA.

Jacquemin

PLATE 6. Valentine III, Emperor of the West, 450–455.

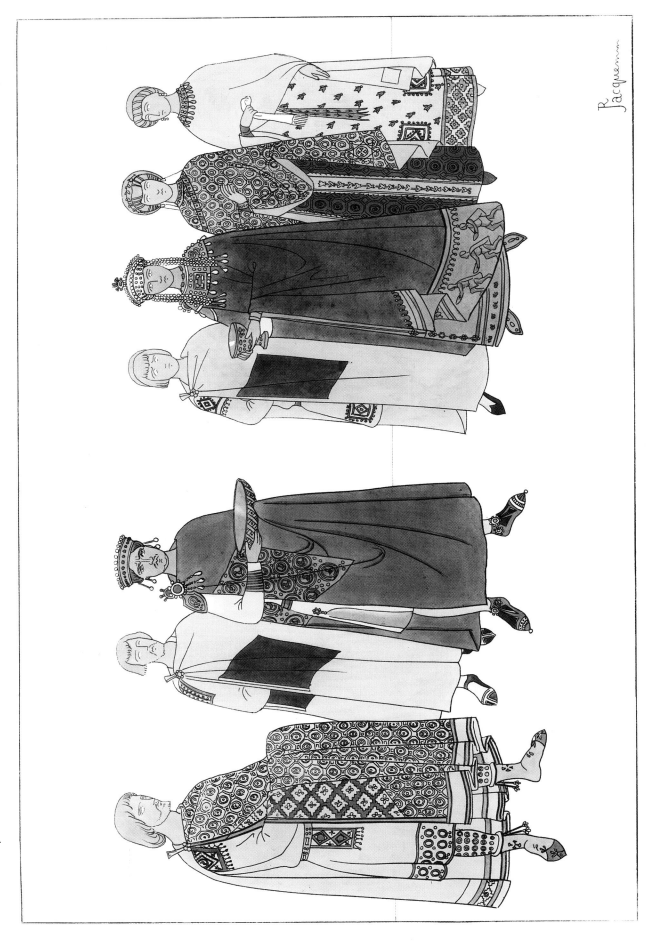

PLATE 7. Emperor Justinian and Empress Theodora with Their Retinues.

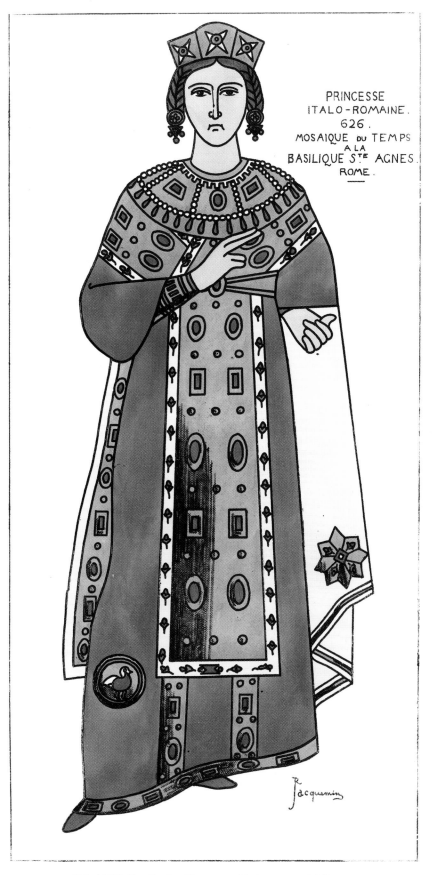

PRINCESSE
ITALO-ROMAINE.
626.
MOSAIQUE ᴅᴜ TEMPS
ᴀ ʟᴀ
BASILIQUE Sᵀᴱ AGNES.
ROME.

PLATE 8. Italo-Roman Princess, 626.

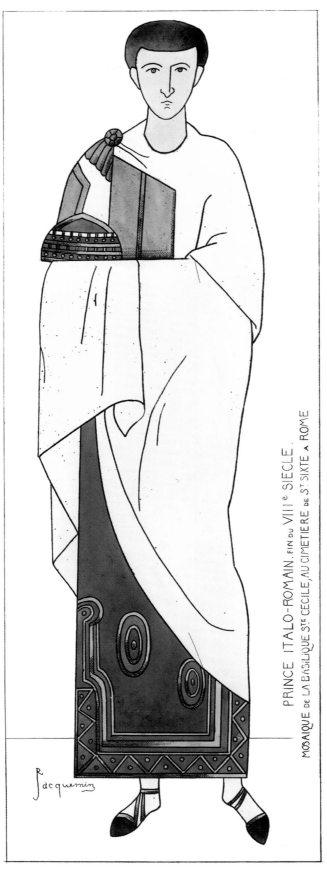

PLATE 9. Italo-Roman Prince. End of the 8th Century.

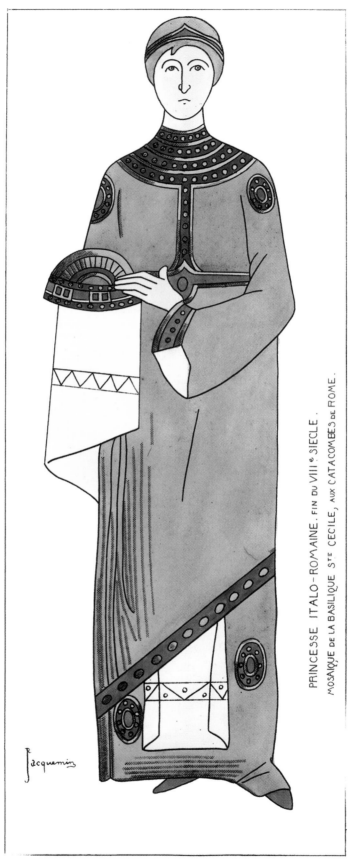

PRINCESSE ITALO-ROMAINE. FIN DU VIIIe SIECLE.
MOSAÏQUE DE LA BASILIQUE Ste CECILE, AUX CATACOMBES DE ROME.

PLATE 10. Italo-Roman Princess. End of the 8th Century.

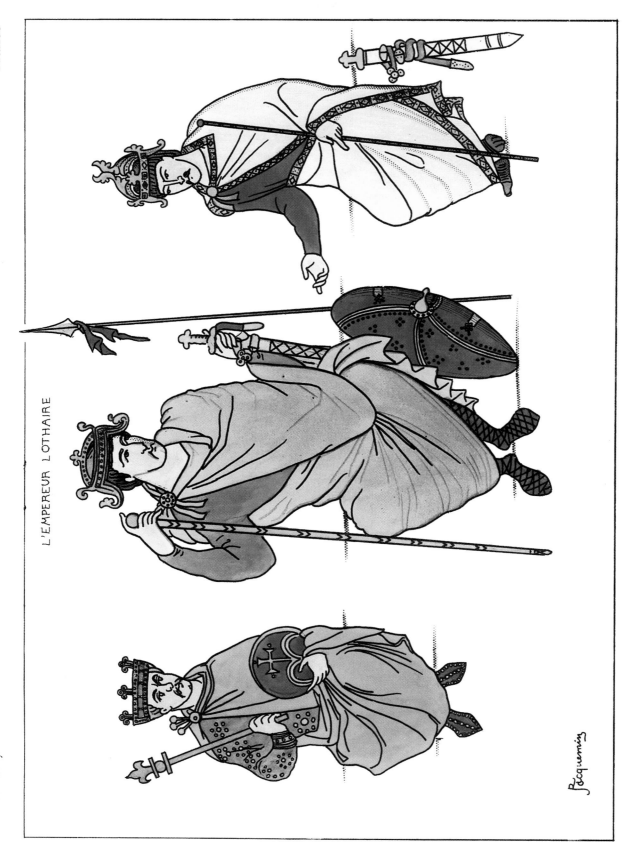

L'EMPEREUR LOTHAIRE

Jacquemin

PLATE 11. Charles the Bald, Emperor of the West, King of the Franks, of Lorraine, etc., 860–75. Emperor Lothair (middle).

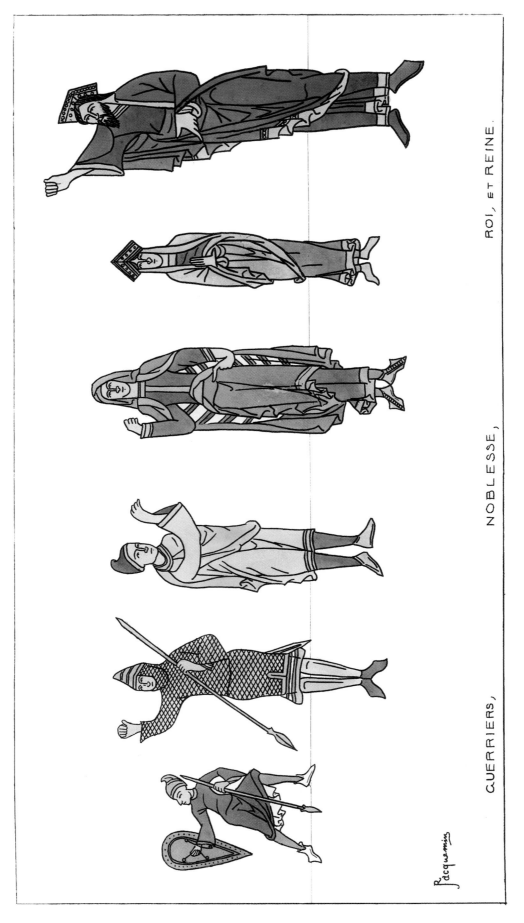

GUERRIERS,   NOBLESSE,   ROI, ET REINE.

PLATE 12. 9th and 10th Century Persons of the Carolingian Epoch. Warriors (left), Nobles (middle), King and Queen (right).

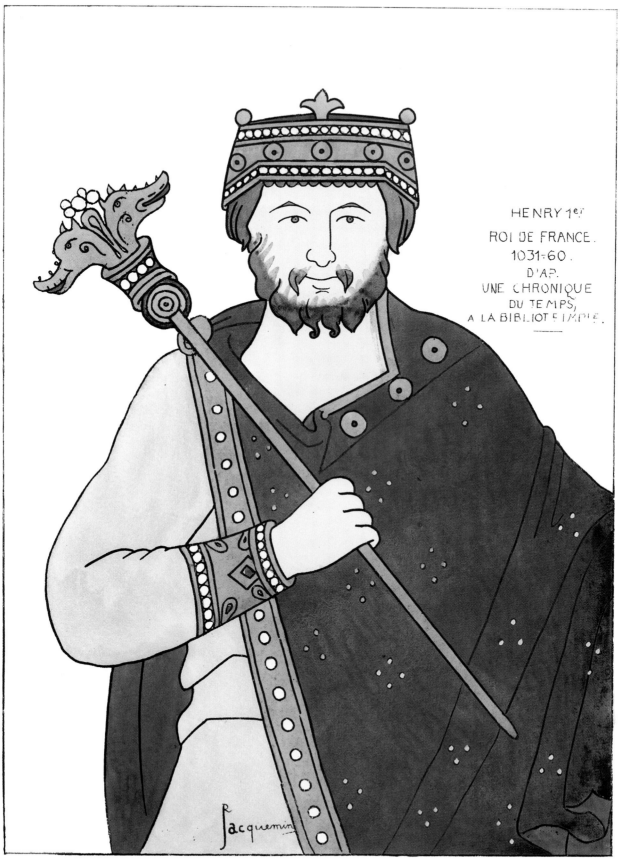

HENRY 1ᵉʳ
ROI DE FRANCE.
1031=60.
D'AP.
UNE CHRONIQUE
DU TEMPS,
A LA BIBLIOTEIMPLE.

PLATE 13. Henry I, King of France, 1031–60.

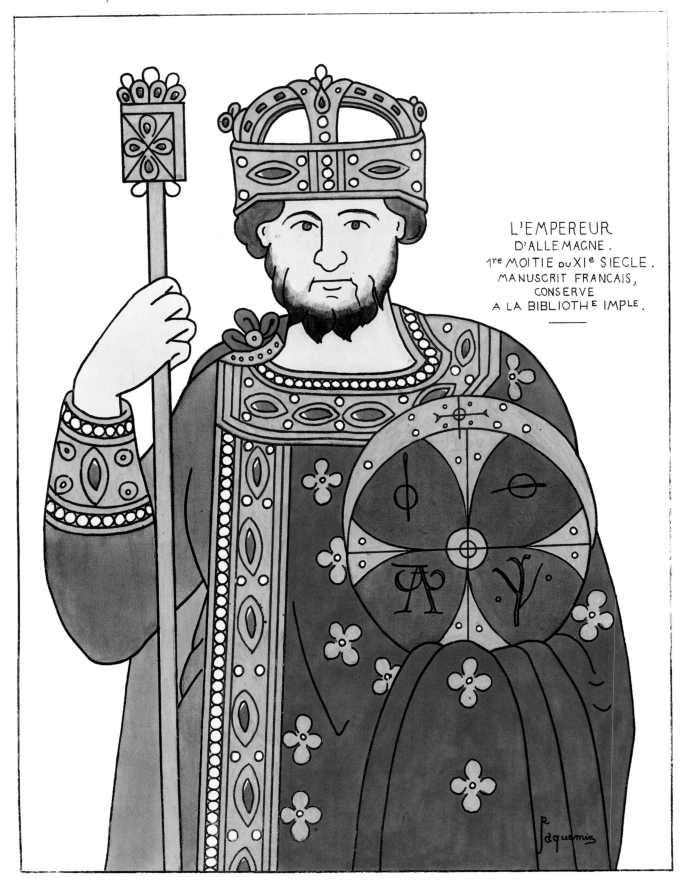

L'EMPEREUR
D'ALLEMAGNE.
1re MOITIE DU XIe SIECLE.
MANUSCRIT FRANCAIS,
CONSERVE
A LA BIBLIOTHe IMPle.

PLATE 14. Emperor of Germany, 1st Half of the 11th Century.

PLATE 15. Norman Warriors of William the Conqueror, 1066.

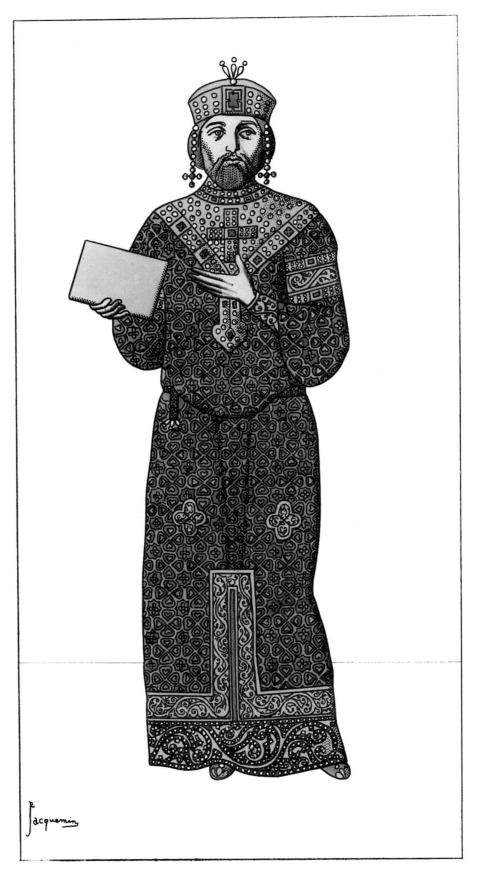

PLATE 16. Nicephore Botaniate, Byzantine Emperor, 1078–81.

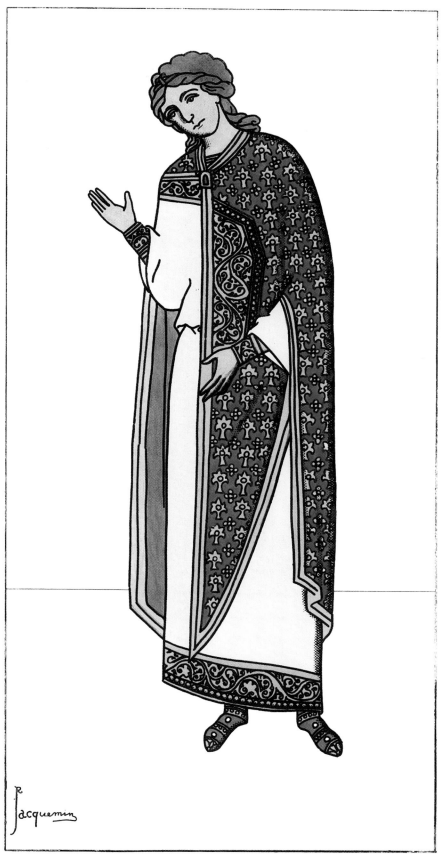

PLATE 17. High Dignitary of the Byzantine Empire, 1078–81.

CHEFS FRANÇAIS.
2me MOITIÉ DU XIme SIÈCLE.
PEINTURES DE MANUSCRITS DU TEMPS
BIBLIOTᴱ IMPᴸᴱ

Jacquemin

PLATE 18. French Chiefs, 2nd Half of the 11th Century.

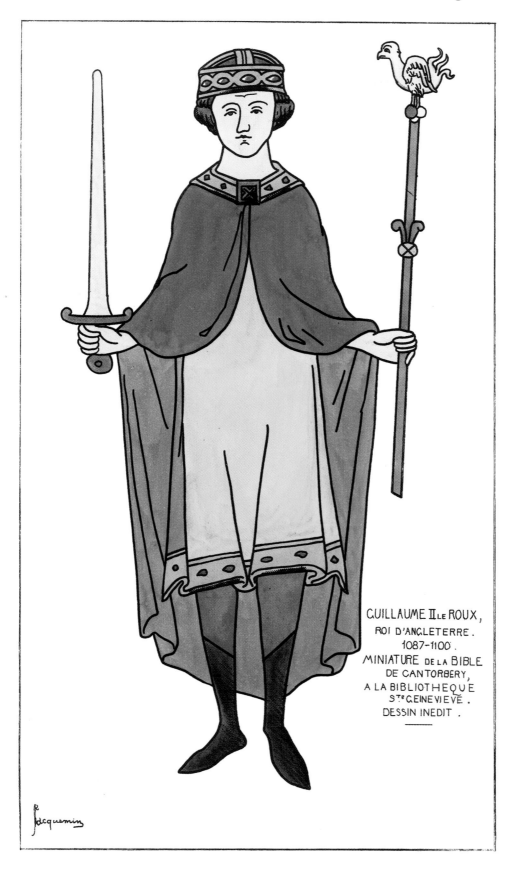

GUILLAUME II LE ROUX,
ROI D'ANGLETERRE.
1087-1100.
MINIATURE DE LA BIBLE
DE CANTORBERY,
A LA BIBLIOTHEQUE
Ste GEINEVIEVE.
DESSIN INEDIT.

PLATE 19. William II ("The Red"), King of England, 1087–1100.

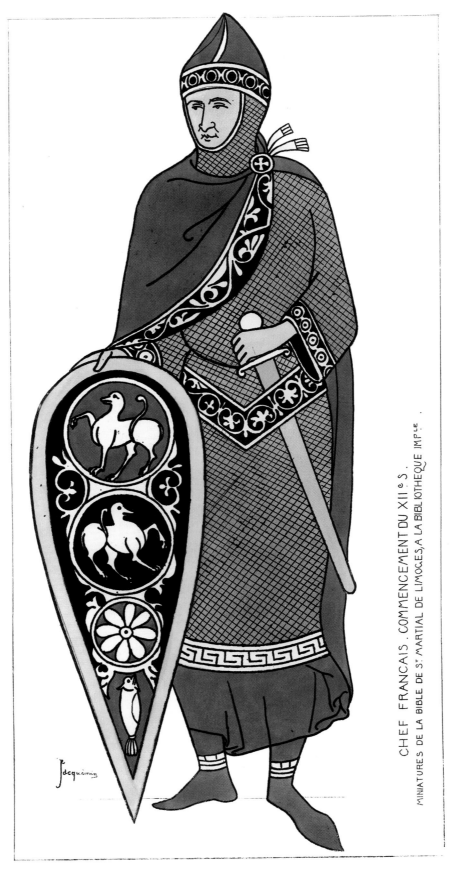

CHEF FRANCAIS . COMMENCEMENT DU XIIᵉ S .
MINIATURES DE LA BIBLE DE Sᵗ MARTIAL DE LIMOGES, A LA BIBLIOTHEQUE IMPᴸᴱ .

PLATE 20. French Chief, Beginning of the 12th Century.

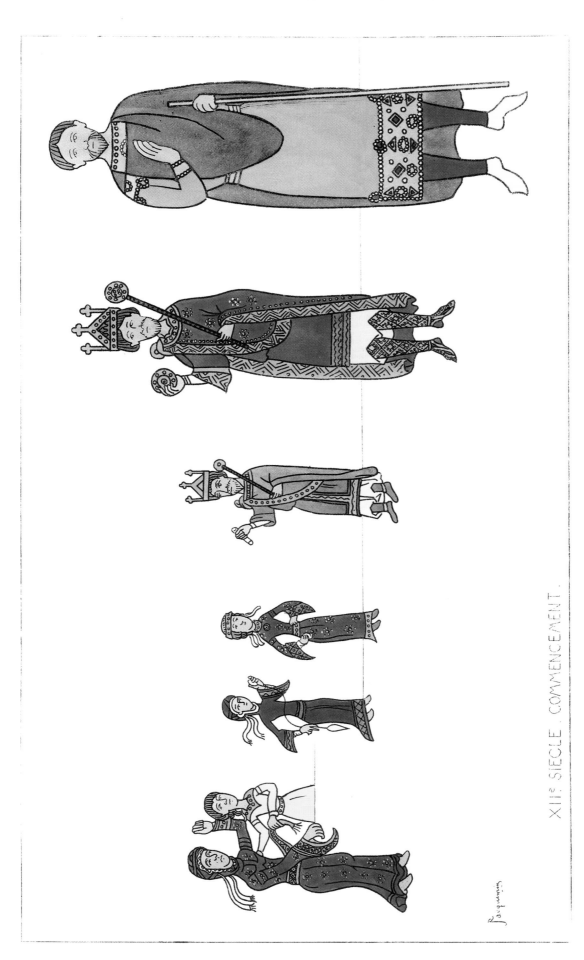

XIIᵉ SIECLE . COMMENCEMENT .

PLATE 21. Monarchs and Middle Class Women of Southern Europe. Beginning of the 12th Century.

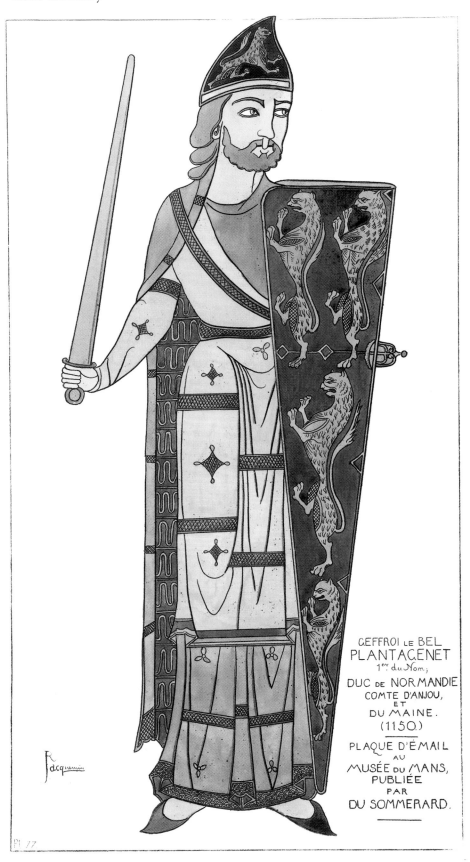

GEFFROI le BEL
PLANTAGENET
1er du Nom;
DUC de NORMANDIE
COMTE D'ANJOU,
et
DU MAINE.
(1150.)

PLAQUE D'ÉMAIL
au
MUSÉE du MANS,
PUBLIÉE
PAR
DU SOMMERARD.

PLATE 22. Geoffrey Plantagenet ("The Fair"), Duke of Normandy, Count of Anjou and of Maine, (1150).

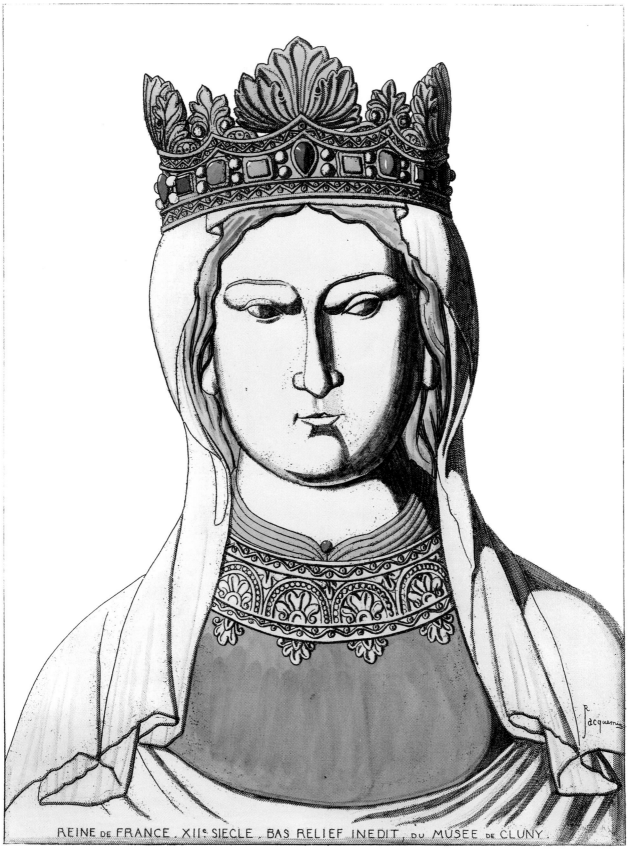

REINE DE FRANCE. XIIᵉ SIECLE. BAS RELIEF INEDIT, DU MUSEE DE CLUNY.

PLATE 23. Queen of France, 12th Century.

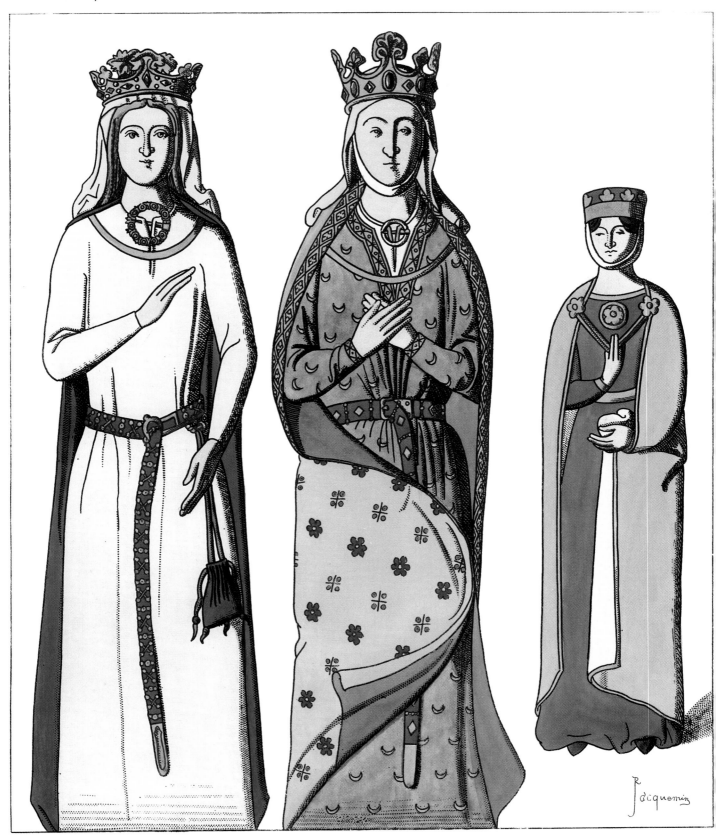

PLATE 24. Bérengère of Navarre, 2nd Wife of King Richard the Lion-Hearted, 1190–1210;
Isabelle of Angouleme, 3rd Wife of King John Sans-Terre, 1200–1220;
Countess of Gleichen, German Lady of the Manor, 1260.

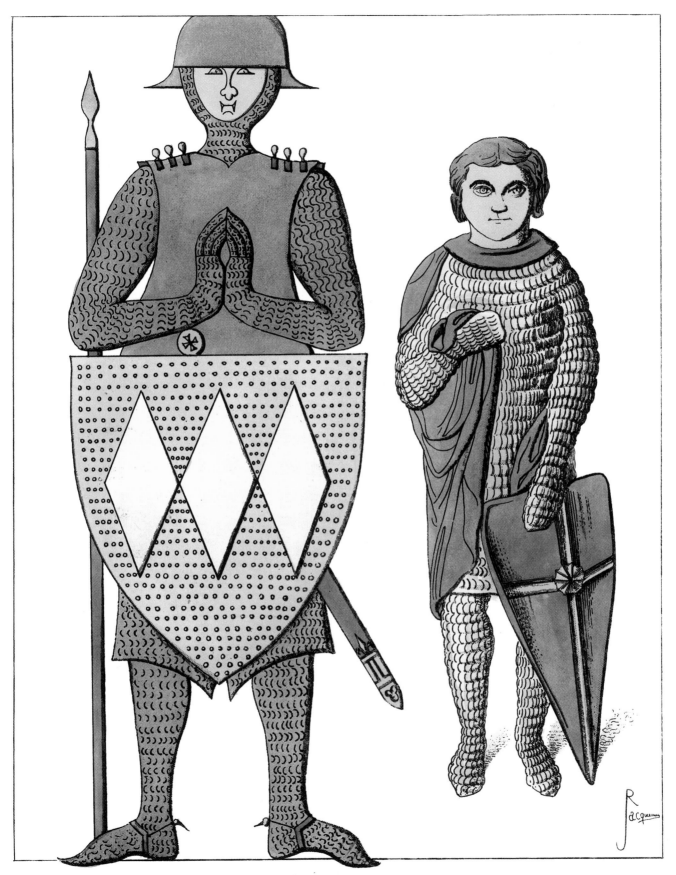

PLATE 25. Brocard of Charpingie, Knight, and Warrior, 1200–1220.

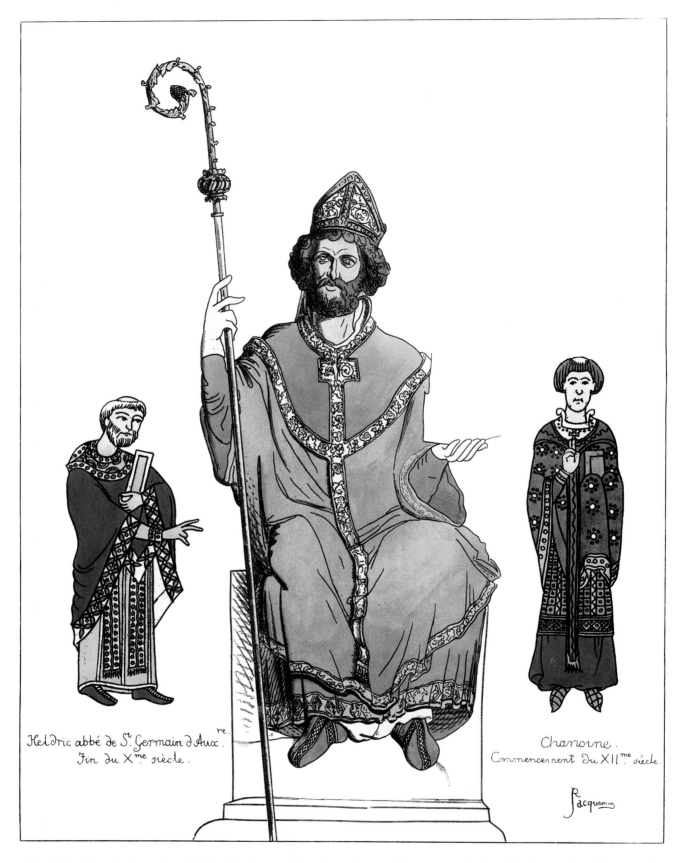

Heldric abbé de St. Germain d'Aux.
Fin du Xme siècle.

Chanoine.
Commencement du XIIme siècle.

Jacquemin

PLATE 26. Bishop in 1247. Shrine of St. Eleuthera. Treasure of the Cathedral of Tournai.

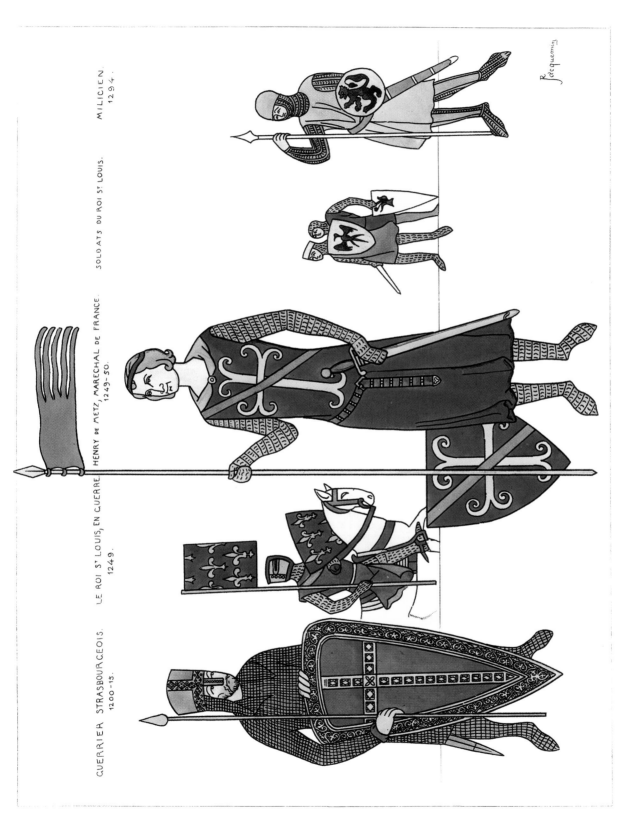

GUERRIER STRASBOURGEOIS.
1200-15.

LE ROI S⁺ LOUIS, EN GUERRE.
1249.

HENRY DE METZ, MARECHAL DE FRANCE.
1249-50.

SOLDATS DU ROI S⁺ LOUIS.

MILICIEN.
1294.

PLATE 27. French Warriors of the 13th Century. Warrior of Strasbourg, 1200–1215 (*left*); King St. Louis at War, 1249 (*second from left*); Henry of Metz, Marshall of France, 1249–1250 (*center*); Soldiers of King St. Louis (*second from right*); Militiaman, 1294 (*far right*).

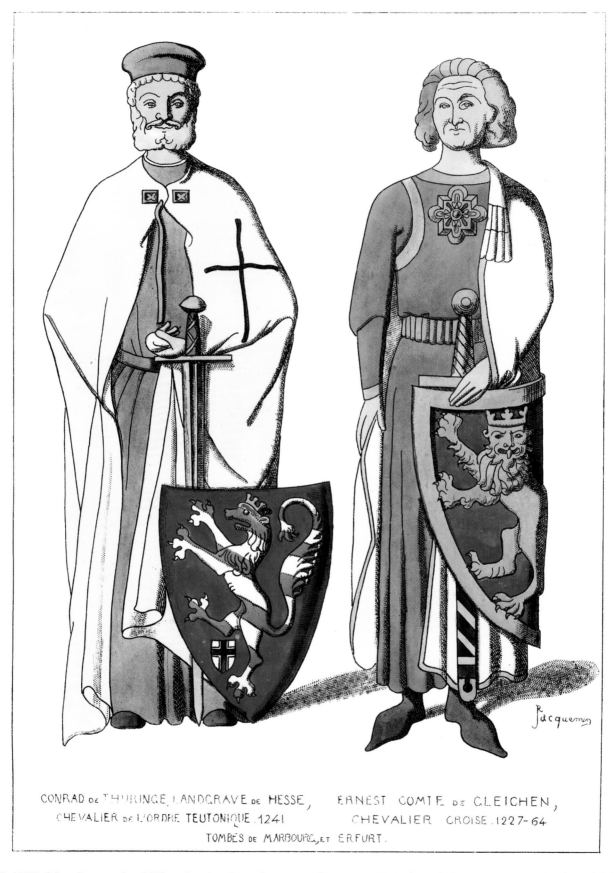

CONRAD de THURINGE, LANDGRAVE de HESSE,   ERNEST COMTE de GLEICHEN,
CHEVALIER de L'ORDRE TEUTONIQUE. 1241   CHEVALIER CROISE. 1227-64.
TOMBES de MARBOURG, et ERFURT.

PLATE 28. Conrad of Thuringia, Landgrave of Hesse, Knight of the Teutonic Order, 1241;
Ernest, Count of Gleichen, Knight of the Crusades, 1227–64.

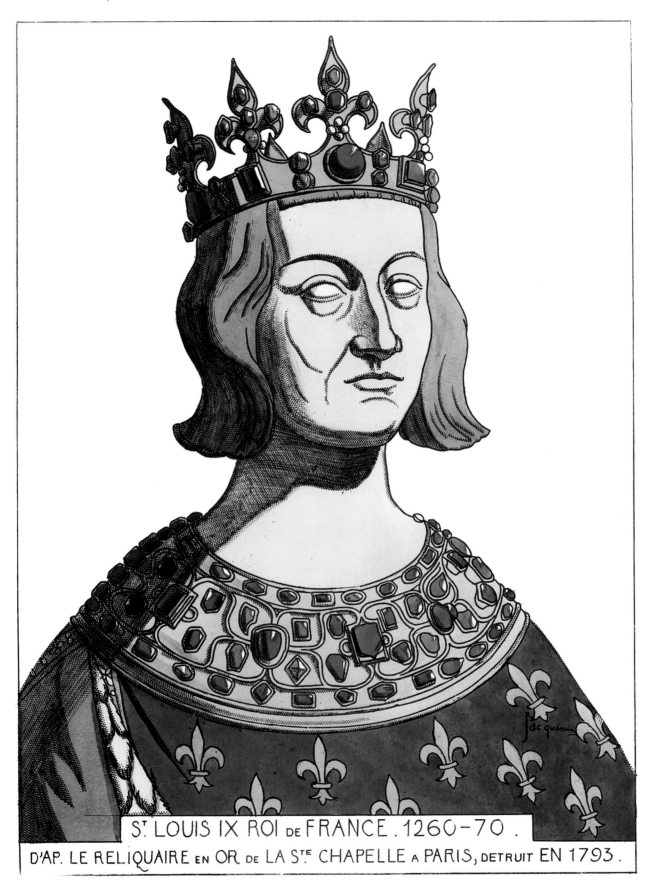

PLATE 29. St. Louis IX, King of France, 1260–70.

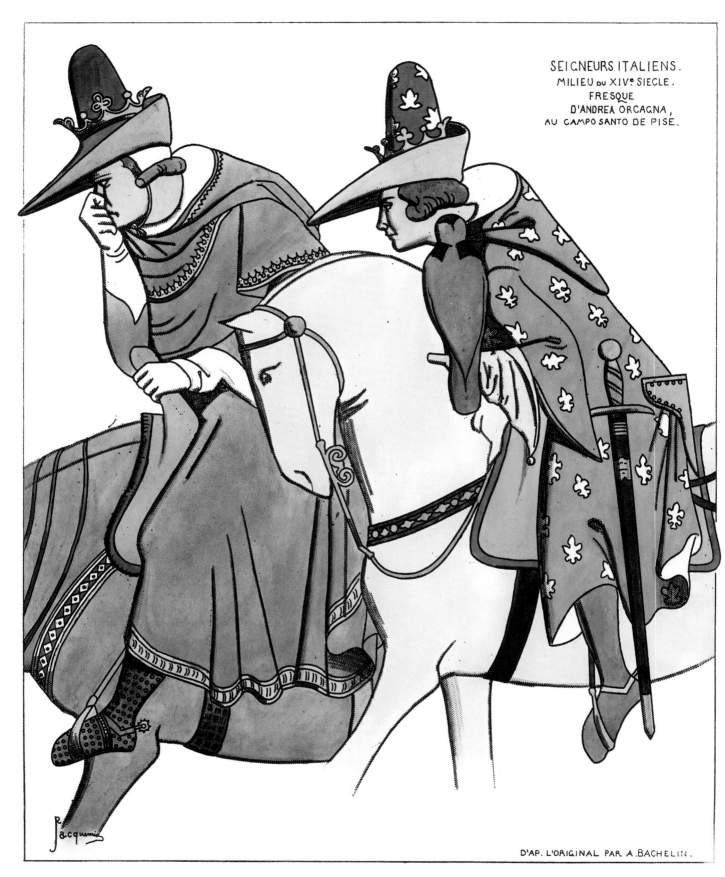

SEIGNEURS ITALIENS.
MILIEU du XIVe SIECLE.
FRESQUE
D'ANDREA ORCAGNA,
AU CAMPO SANTO DE PISE.

D'AP. L'ORIGINAL PAR A. BACHELIN.

PLATE 30. Italian Lords, Middle of the 14th Century.

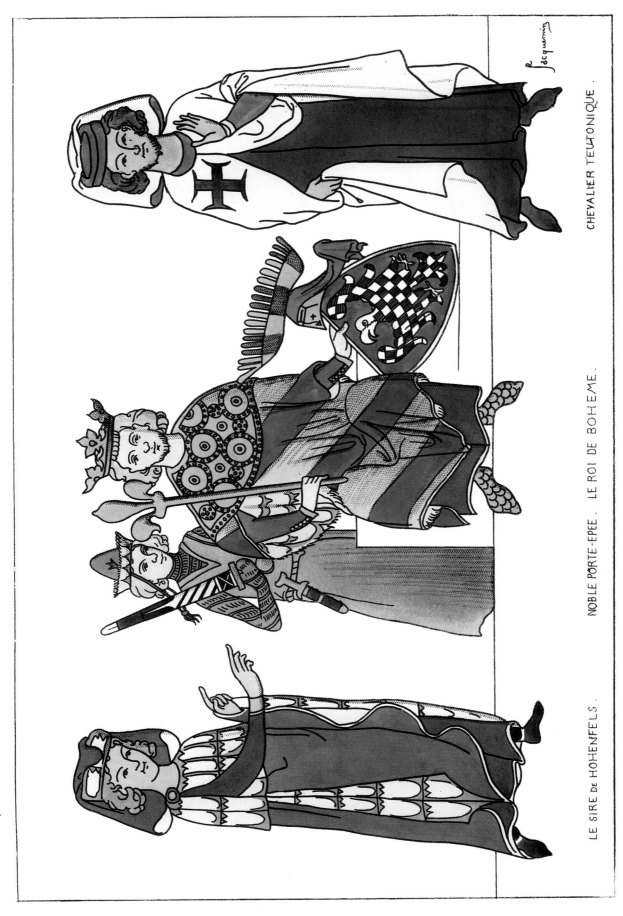

LE SIRE DE HOHENFELS.

NOBLE PORTE-EPEE. LE ROI DE BOHEME.

CHEVALIER TEUTONIQUE.

PLATE 31. German Personages. Middle of the 14th Century. Lord of Hohenfels (*left*); Noble's sword-carrier (*second from left*); King of Bohemia (*second from right*); Teutonic Knight (*far right*).

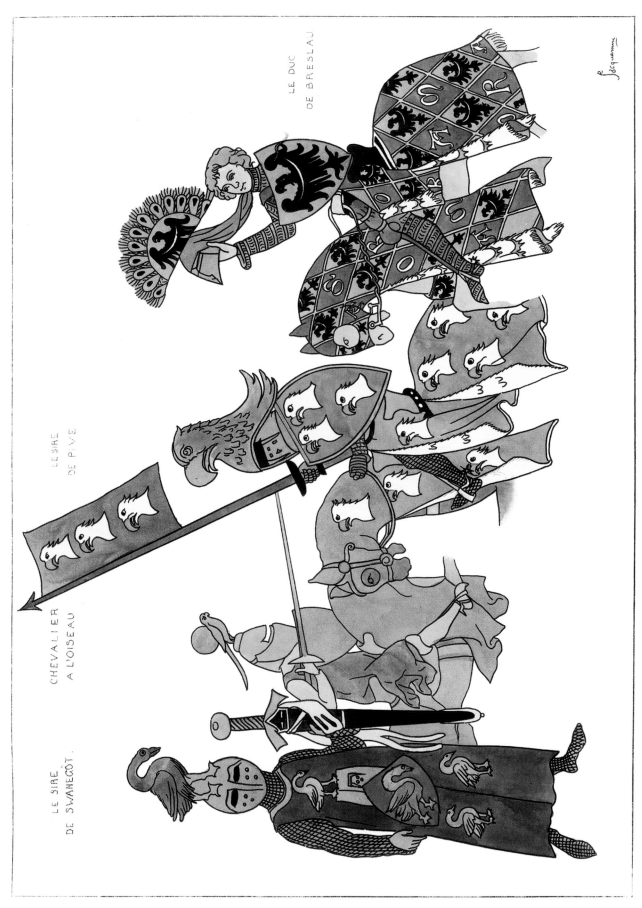

LE SIRE
DE SWANEGÖT.

CHEVALIER
A L'OISEAU

LE SIRE
DE PIVE

LE DUC
DE BRESLAU

PLATE 32. German Lords at a Tournament. (Middle of the 14th Century). Lord of Swanegöt (*left*); Bird Knight (*second from left*); Lord of Wine (*second from right*); Duke of Breslau (*far right*).

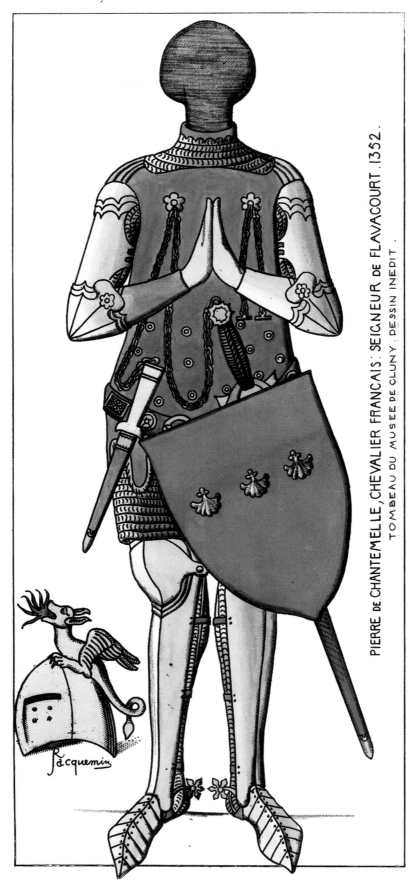

PIERRE DE CHANTEMELLE, CHEVALIER FRANCAIS : SEIGNEUR DE FLAVACOURT. 1352.
TOMBEAU DU MUSÉE DE CLUNY. DESSIN INÉDIT.

PLATE 33. Pierre de Chantemelle, French Knight: Lord of Flavacourt, 1352.

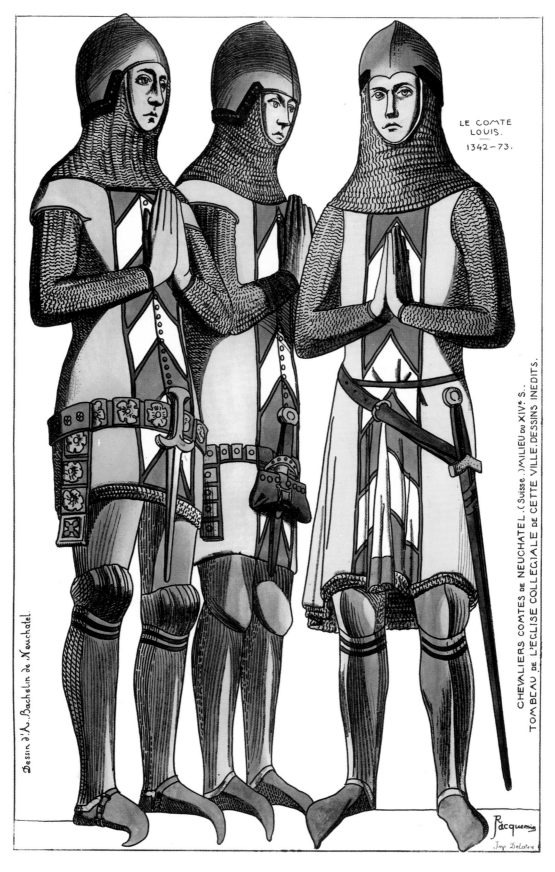

LE COMTE
LOUIS.
—
1342–73.

Dessin d'A. Bachelin de Neuchatel.

CHEVALIERS COMTES de NEUCHATEL. (Suisse.) MILIEU du XIVᵉ S.
TOMBEAU de L'EGLISE COLLEGIALE de CETTE VILLE. DESSINS INEDITS.

Jacquemin
Imp Delatre

PLATE 34. Knight-Counts of Neuchatel (Swiss). Middle of 14th Century.
Count Louis, 1342–73 (*far right*).

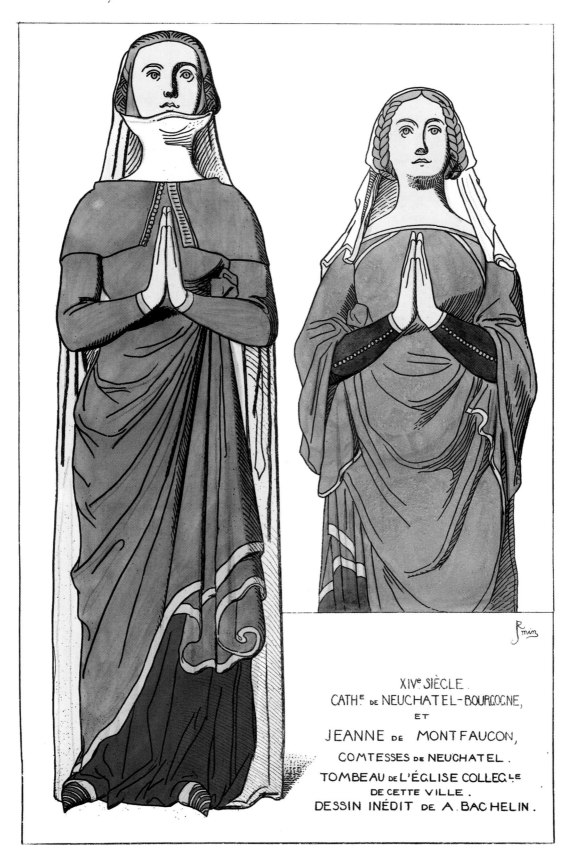

XIVᵉ SIÈCLE.
CATHᵉ ᴅᴇ NEUCHATEL-BOURGOGNE,
ᴇᴛ
JEANNE ᴅᴇ MONTFAUCON,
COMTESSES ᴅᴇ NEUCHATEL.
TOMBEAU ᴅᴇ L'ÉGLISE COLLEGᴸᴇ
ᴅᴇ CETTE VILLE.
DESSIN INÉDIT ᴅᴇ A. BACHELIN.

PLATE 35. 14th Century. Catherine of Neuchatel-Bourgogne and Jeanne of Montfaucon,
Countesses of Neuchatel.

14th Century

Italy

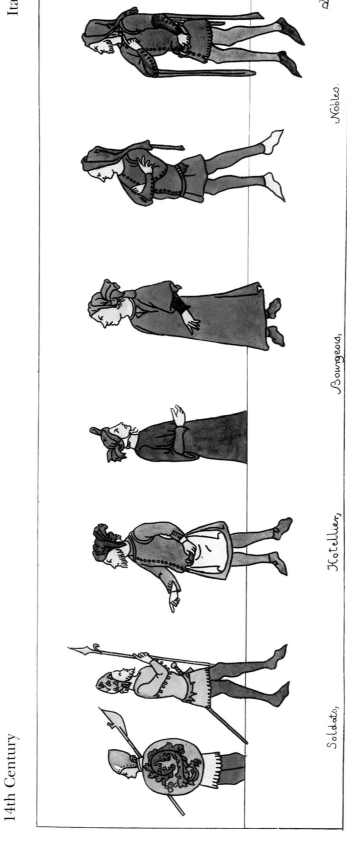

Soldats,   Hotellier,   Bourgeois,   Nobles.

Bedmann

PLATE 36. Italian Personages of the 14th Century. *Left to right:* Soldiers, Innkeeper, Commoners, Nobles.

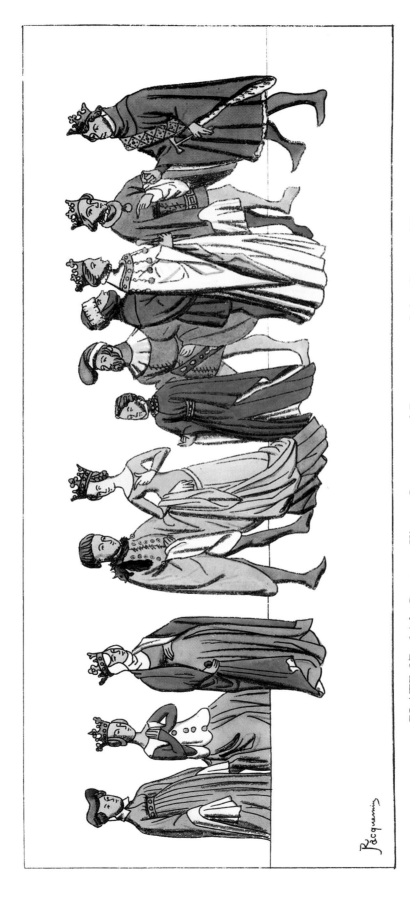

PLATE 37. 14th Century. Kings, Queens, and Personages of the Court of France.

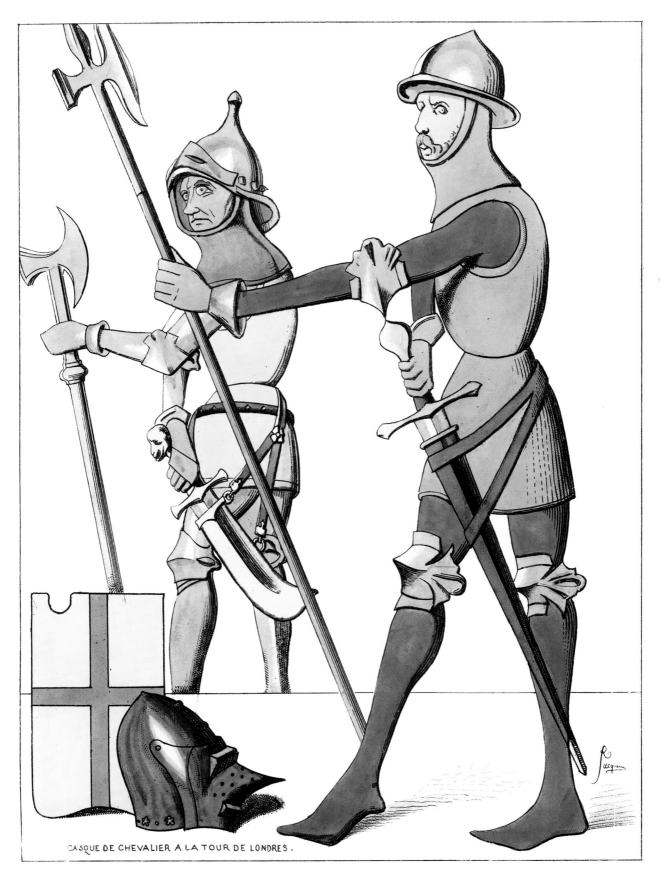

CASQUE DE CHEVALIER A LA TOUR DE LONDRES.

PLATE 38. Men-at-Arms. Epoch of King John. Knight's Helmet at the Tower of London.

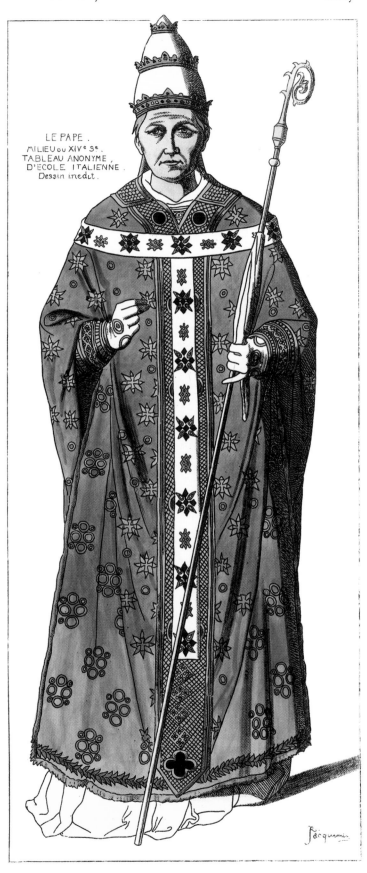

LE PAPE.
MILIEU ou XIVᵉ Sᵉ.
TABLEAU ANONYME,
D'ECOLE ITALIENNE.
Dessin inedit.

PLATE 39. Pope. Middle of the 14th Century.

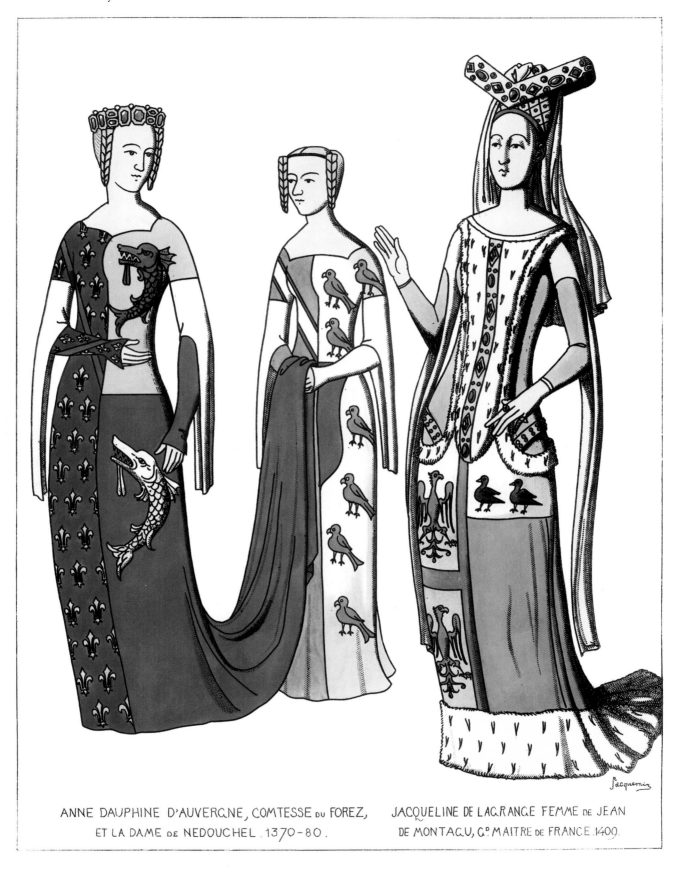

ANNE DAUPHINE D'AUVERGNE, COMTESSE DU FOREZ, ET LA DAME DE NEDOUCHEL . 1370-80 .

JACQUELINE DE LAGRANGE FEMME DE JEAN DE MONTAGU, G° MAITRE DE FRANCE .1409.

PLATE 40. Anne, Dauphine of Auvergne, Countess of Forez, and the Lady of Nedouchel, 1370–80. (*right*) Jacqueline of LaGrange, Wife of Jean de Montagu, Grand Master of France, 1409.

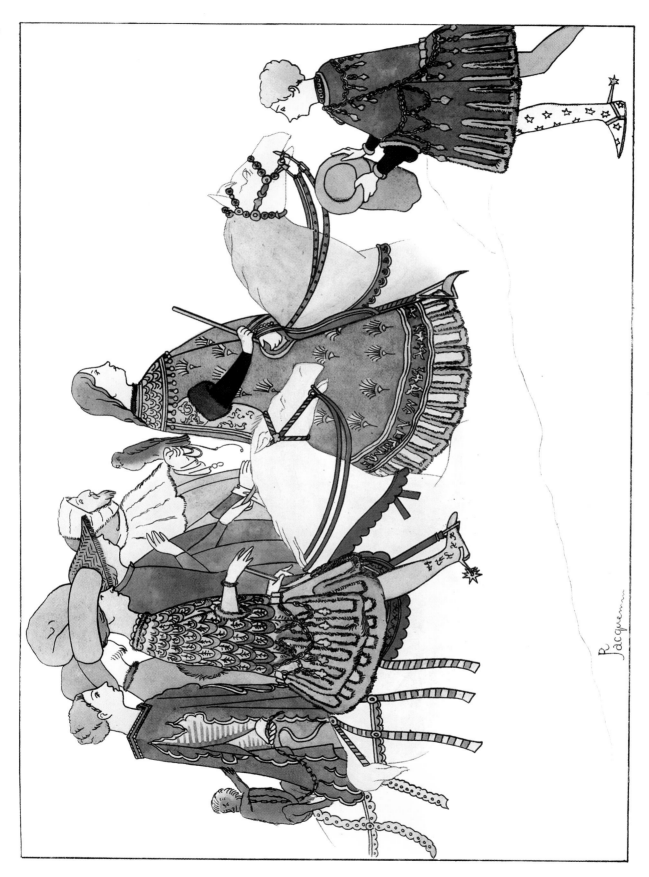

PLATE 41. Visiting Cavalcade of a Lord.

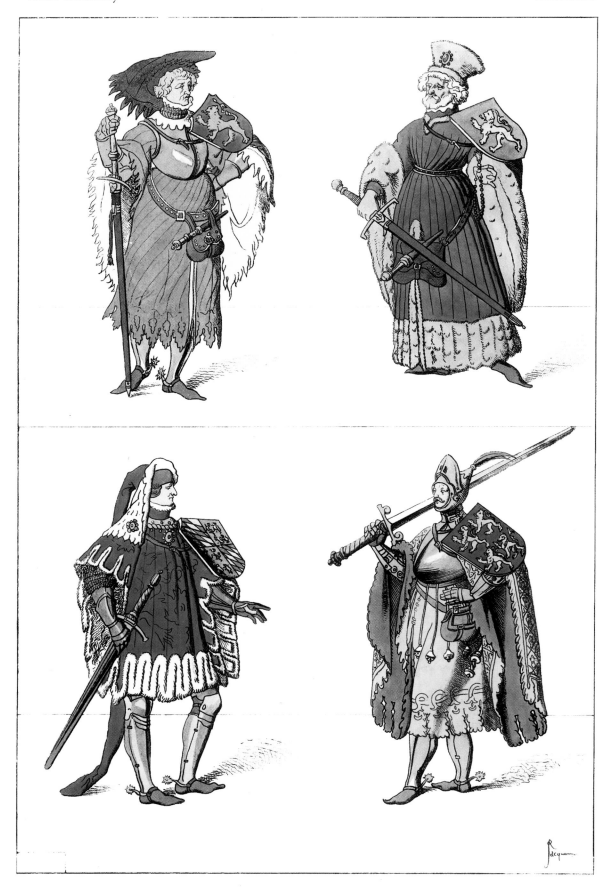

PLATE 42. 15th Century. Counts of Holland and Flanders.

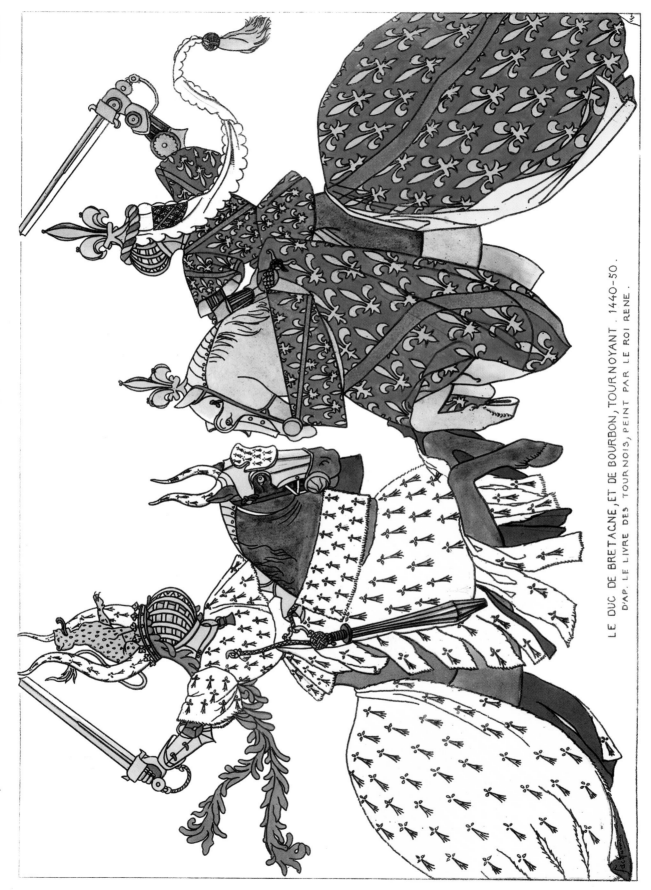

LE DUC DE BRETAGNE, ET DE BOURBON, TOURNOYANT. 1440-50.
D'AP. LE LIVRE DES TOURNOIS, PEINT PAR LE ROI RENE.

PLATE 43. The Dukes of Brittany and Bourbon in a Tournament, 1440-50.

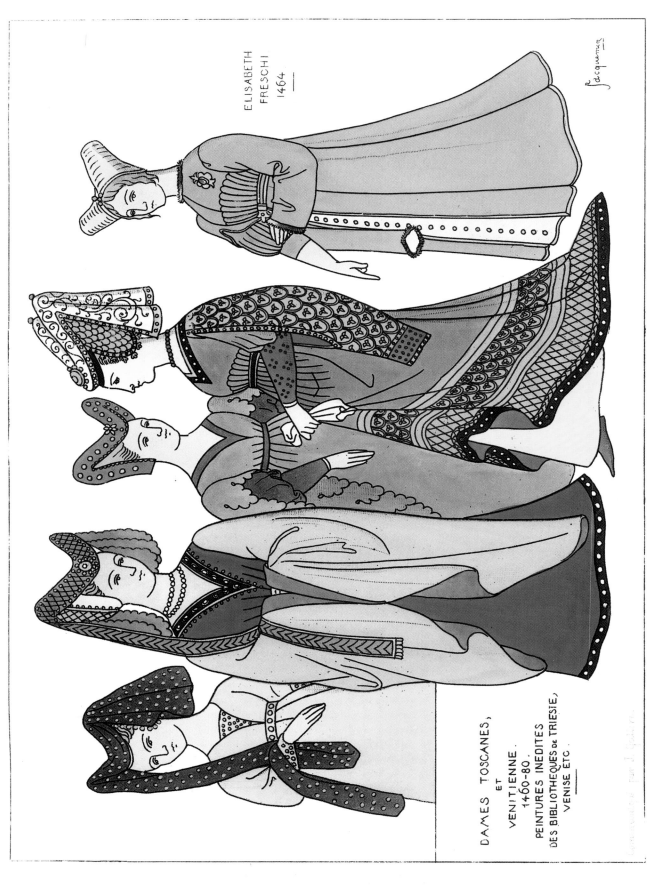

ELISABETH
FRESCHI
1464

DAMES TOSCANES,
ET
VENITIENNE.
1460-80.
PEINTURES INEDITES
DES BIBLIOTHEQUES DE TRIESTE,
VENISE ETC.

PLATE 44. Tuscan and Venetian Ladies, 1460–1480. Elisabeth Freschi, 1464.

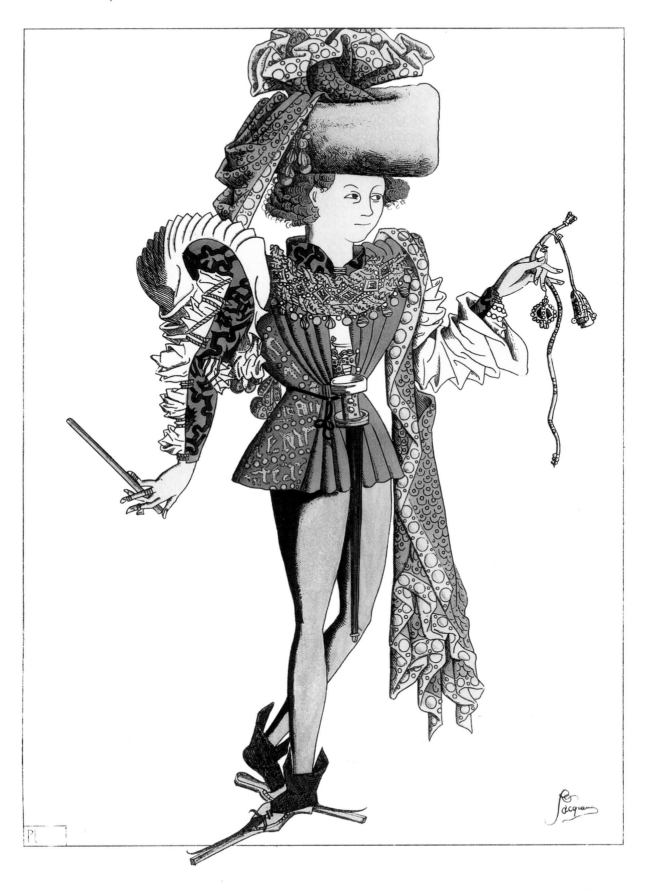

PLATE 45. Elegant Youth, 1480.

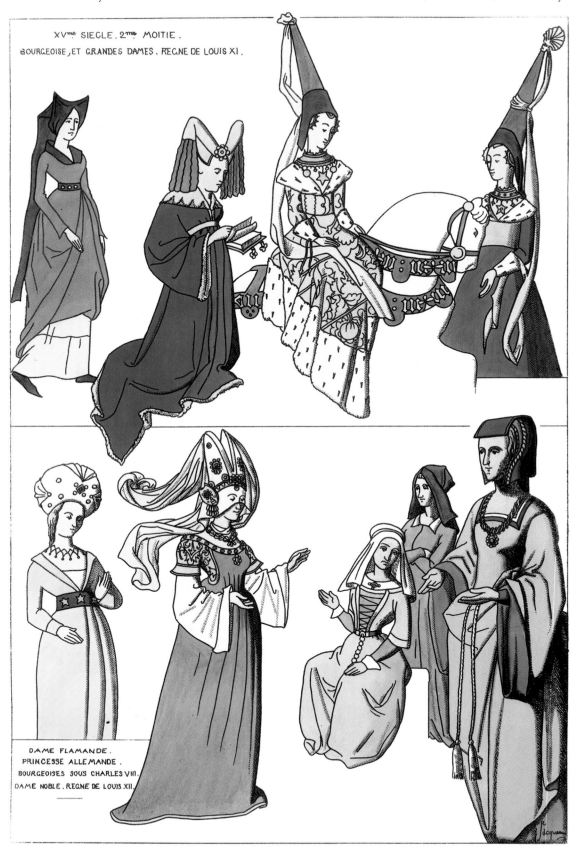

PLATE 46. (*top*) 15th Century, 2nd Half. Middle Class Women and Great Ladies, Reign of Louis XI. (*bottom-left to right*) Flemish Lady, German Princess, Middle Class Women in the Time of Charles VIII, Noble Lady, Reign of Louis XII.

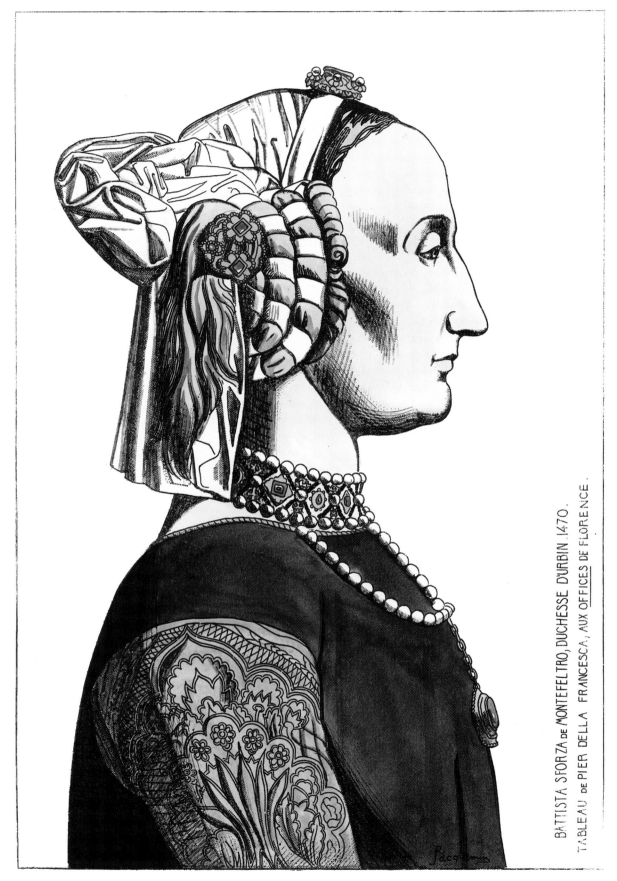

BATTISTA SFORZA DE MONTEFELTRO, DUCHESSE D'URBIN 1470.

TABLEAU DE PIER DELLA FRANCESCA, AUX OFFICES DE FLORENCE.

PLATE 47. Battista Sforza of Montefeltro, Duchess of Urbino, 1470.

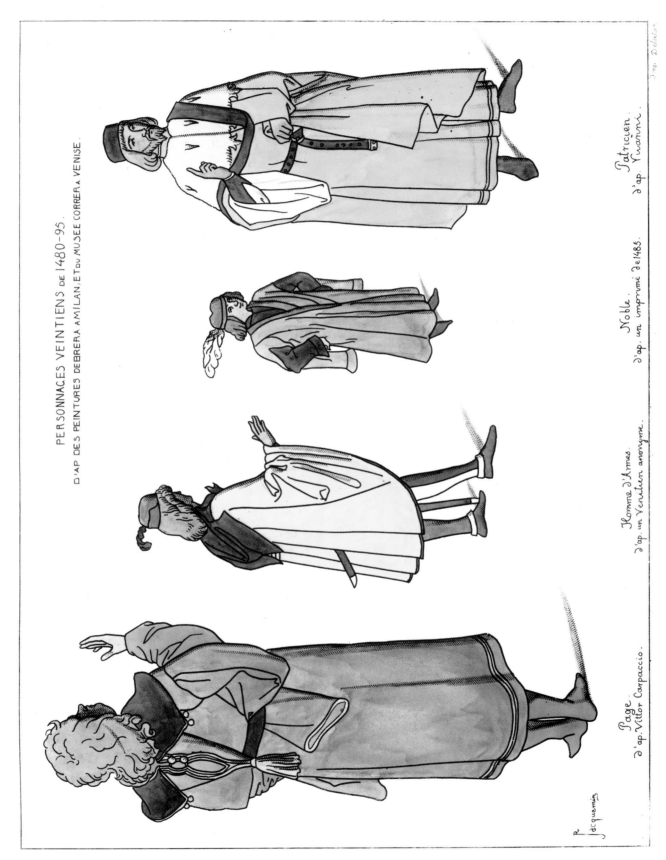

PERSONNAGES VÉNITIENS de 1480-95.
D'AP DES PEINTURES DEBRERA AMILAN, ET DU MUSÉE CORRERA VENISE.

Page.
d'ap. Vittor Carpaccio.

Homme d'Armes.
d'ap. un Vénitien anonyme.

Noble.
d'ap. un imprimé de 1485.

Patricien.
d'ap. Yuanini.

PLATE 48. Venetian Personages of 1480-95. *Left to right:* Page, Man-of-Arms, Noble, Patrician.

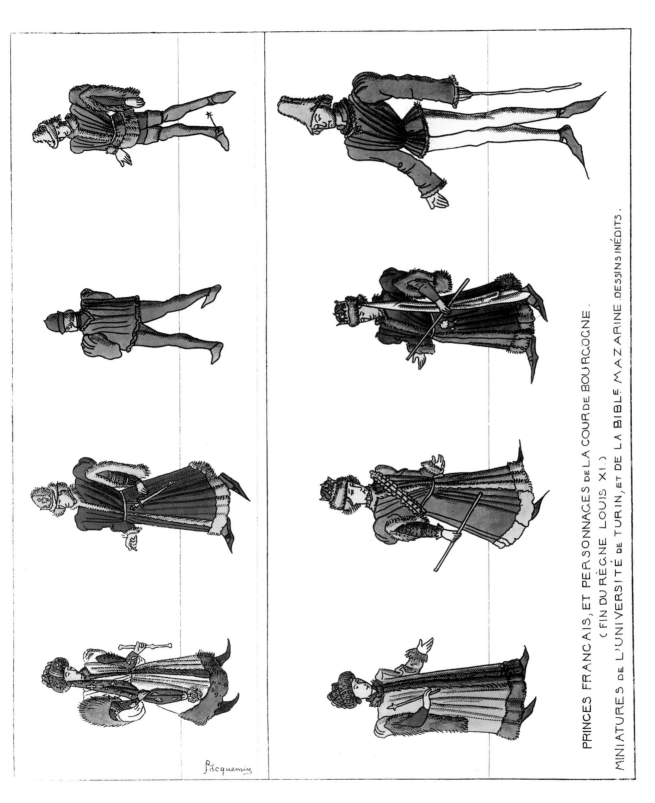

PRINCES FRANCAIS, ET PERSONNAGES DE LA COUR DE BOURGOGNE.

(FIN DU RÈGNE LOUIS XI.)

MINIATURES DE L'UNIVERSITÉ DE TURIN, ET DE LA BIBLE MAZARINE. DESSINS INÉDITS.

PLATE 49. French Princes and Personages of the Court of Burgundy (End of the Reign of Louis XI).

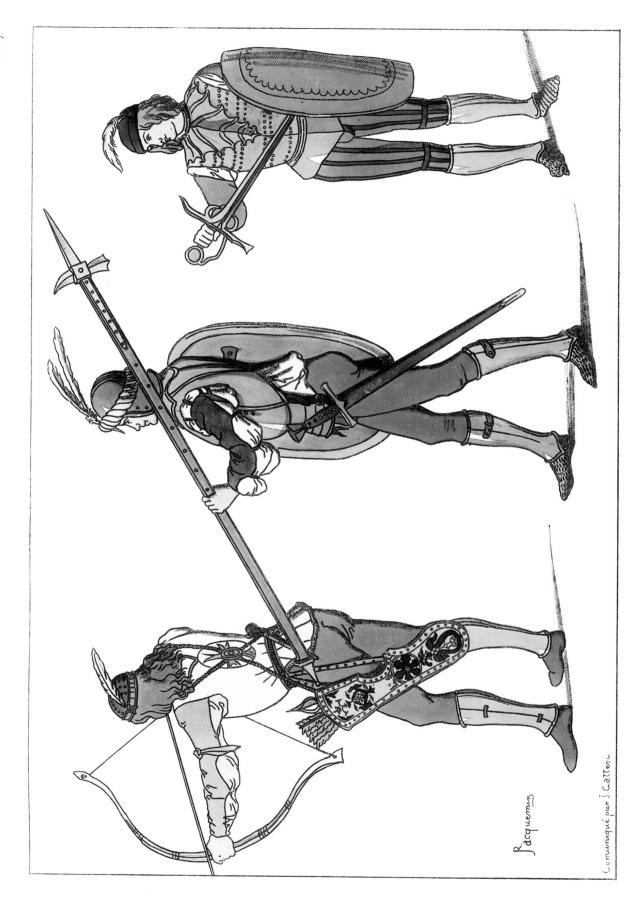

Jacquemin

Comuniqué par J. Catteri

PLATE 50. Venetian Men-at-Arms. End of the 15th Century.

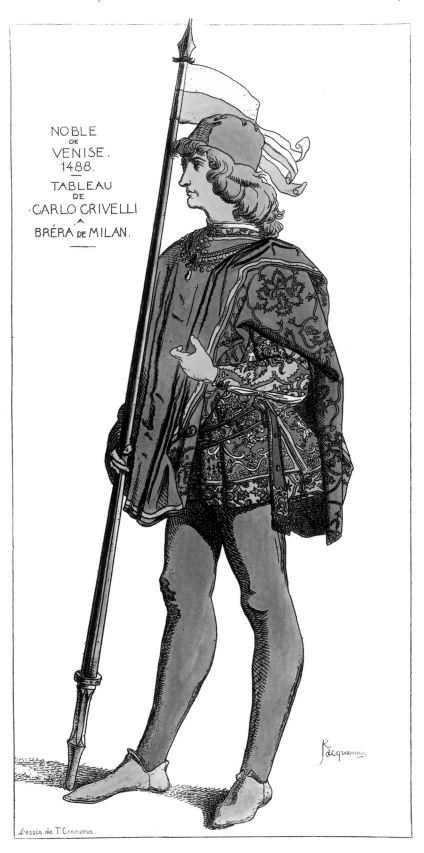

NOBLE
DE
VENISE.
1488.

TABLEAU
DE
·CARLO CRIVELLI
^
BRÉRA DE MILAN.

PLATE 51. Venetian Noble, 1488.

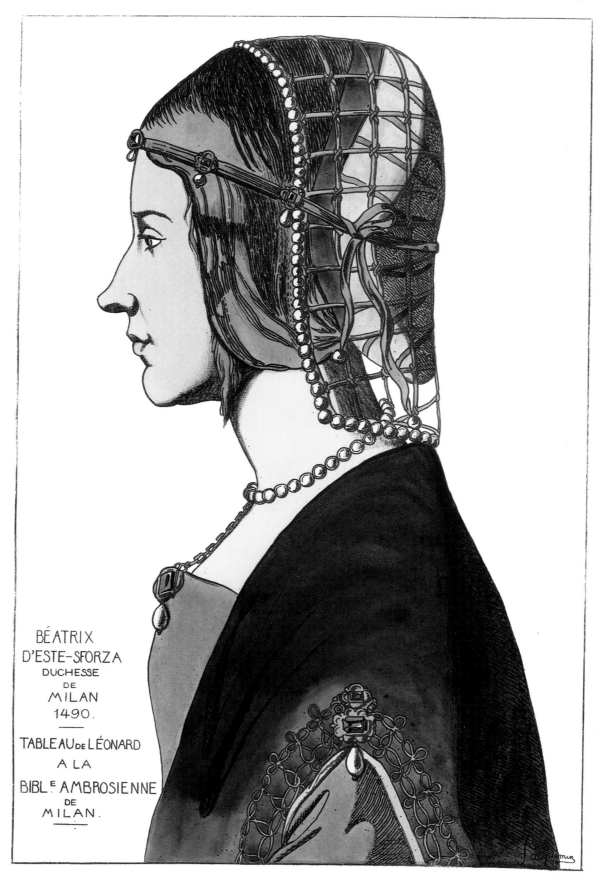

BÉATRIX
D'ESTE-SFORZA
DUCHESSE
DE
MILAN
1490.

TABLEAU DE LÉONARD
A LA
BIBLᴱ AMBROSIENNE
DE
MILAN.

PLATE 52. Beatrice D'Este-Sforza, Duchess of Milan, 1490.

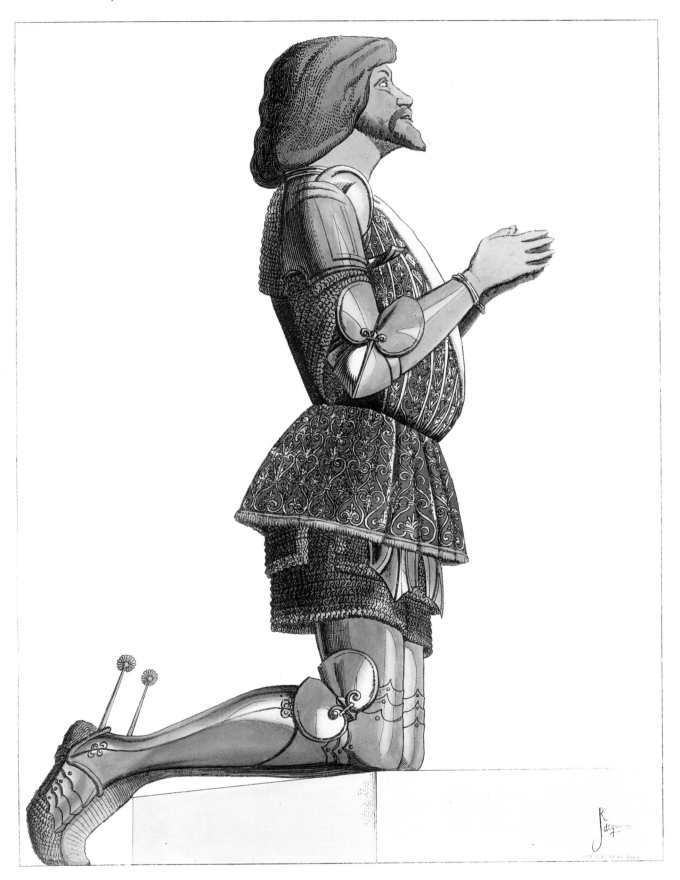

PLATE 53. Jean-François de Gonzague, Marquis of Mantua (1495).

PLATE 54. Noblemen and Falconer, Venetian Costumes, 15th Century.

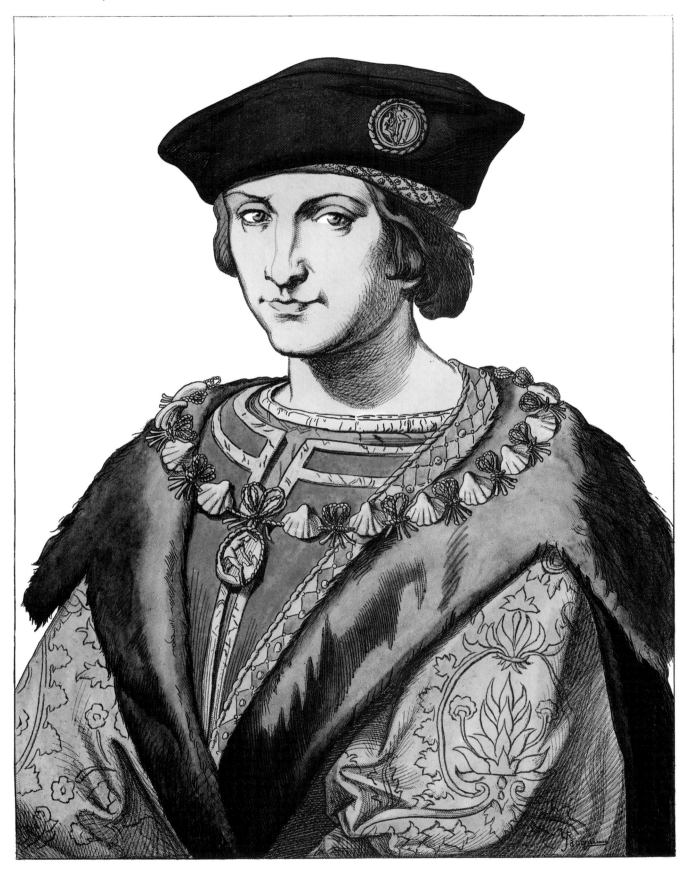

PLATE 55. Charles VIII, King of France (1494–98).

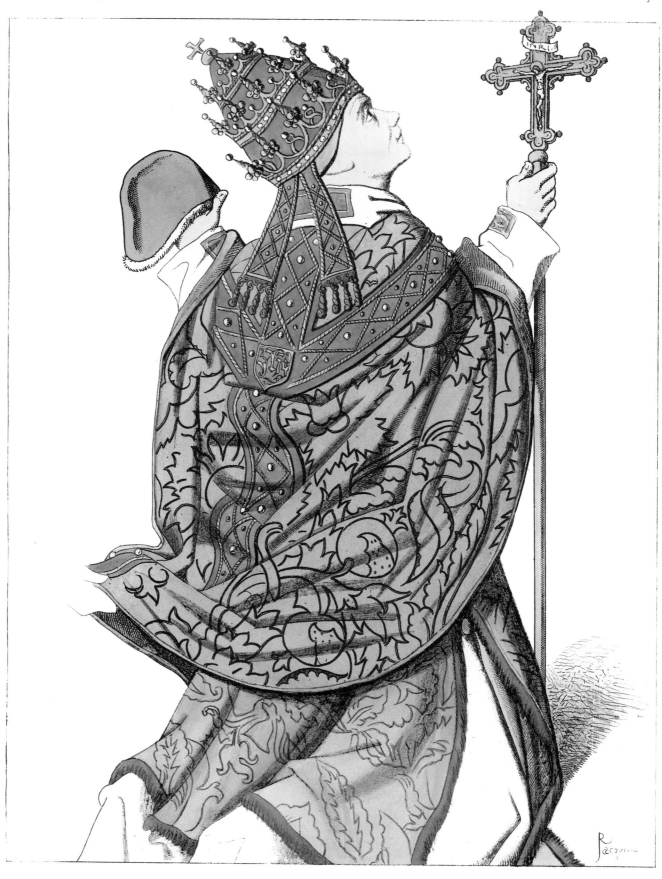

PLATE 56. The Pope Officiating.

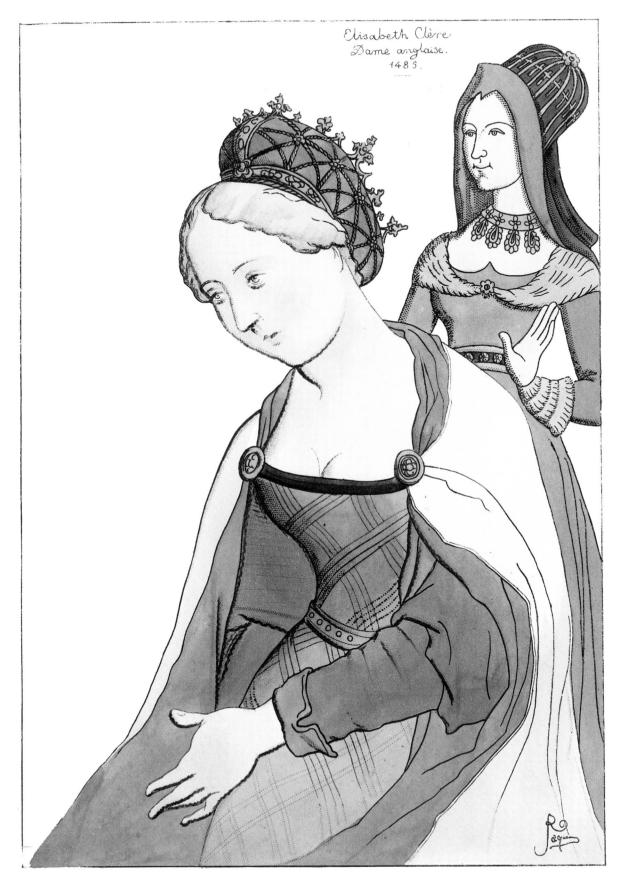

Elisabeth Clère
Dame anglaise.
1485.

PLATE 57. Flemish Noblewoman, 1495. (*At rear*) Elizabeth Clère, English Lady, 1485.

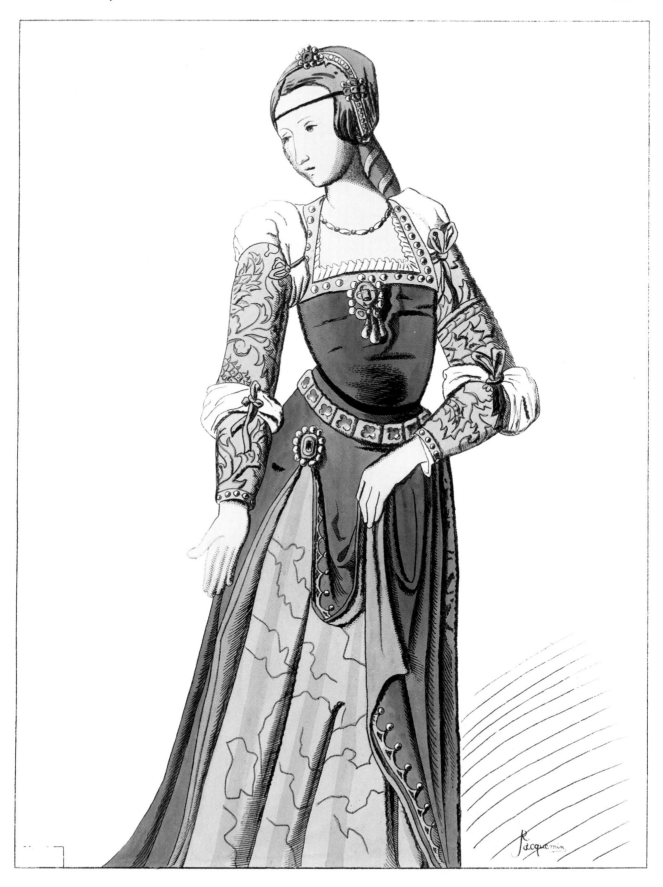

PLATE 58. Flemish Noblewoman, 1500–1510.

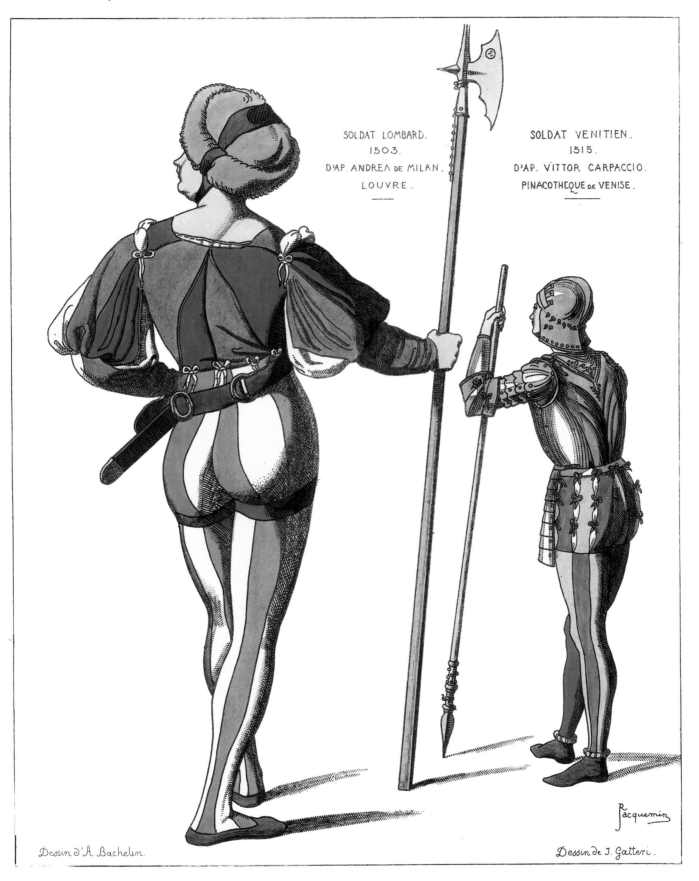

SOLDAT LOMBARD.
1503.
D'AP. ANDREA DE MILAN.
LOUVRE.

SOLDAT VENITIEN.
1515.
D'AP. VITTOR CARPACCIO.
PINACOTHEQUE DE VENISE.

Dessin d'A. Bachelin.

Dessin de I. Gatteri.

PLATE 59. Lombard Soldier, 1503; Venetian Soldier, 1515.

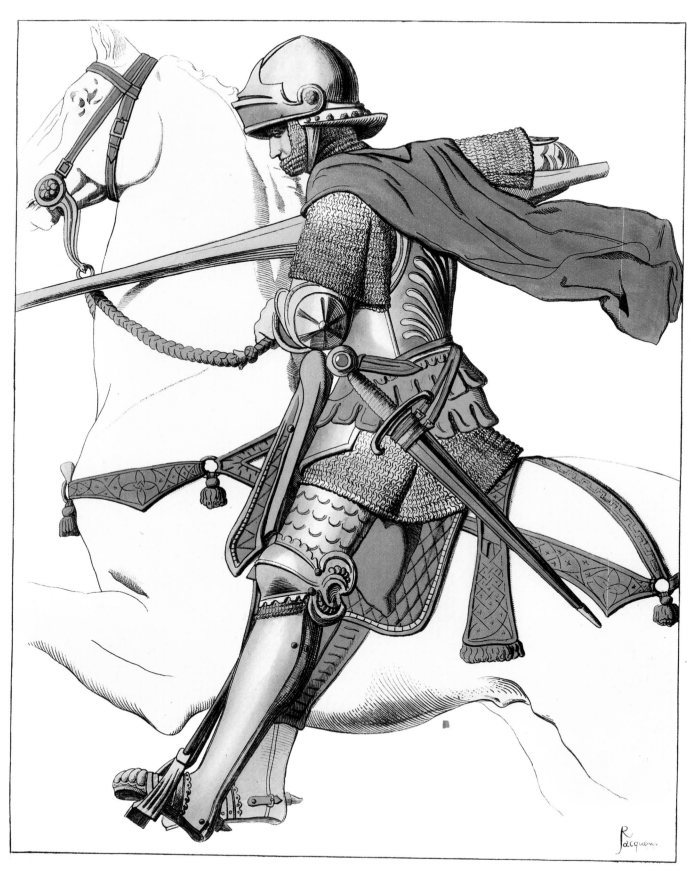

PLATE 60. French Knight Jousting, 1508.

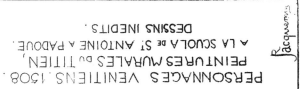

PERSONNAGES VENITIENS 1508.
PEINTURES MURALES DU TITIEN,
A LA SCUOLA DE ST ANTOINE A PADOUE.
DESSINS INEDITS.

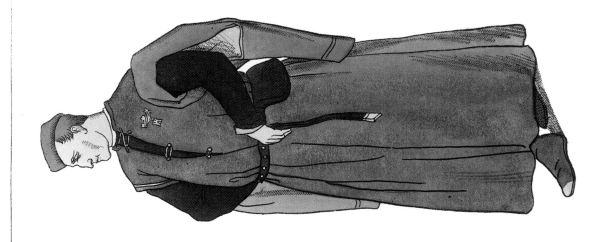

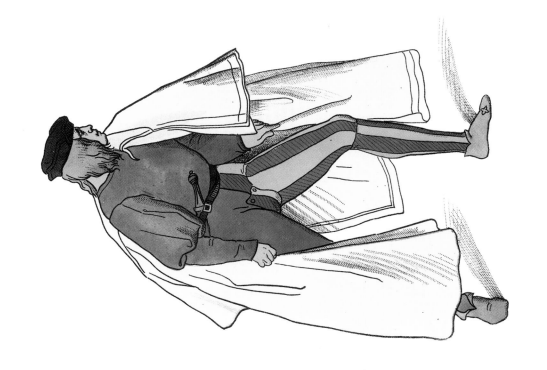

Communiqué par J. GATTERI.

PLATE 61. Venetian Personages, 1508.

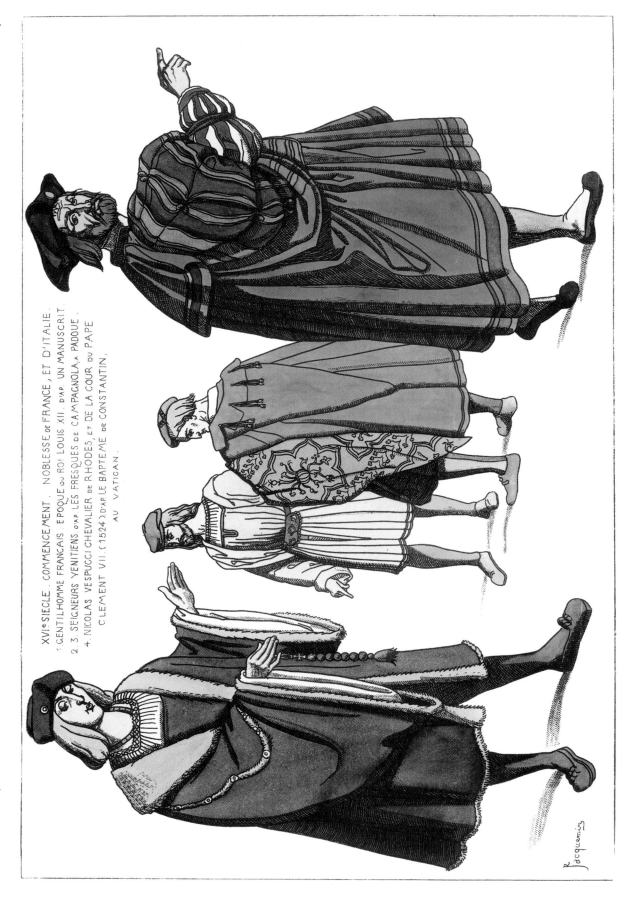

XVIᵉ SIECLE . COMMENCEMENT . NOBLESSE ᴅᴇ FRANCE , ET D'ITALIE .
1. GENTILHOMME FRANÇAIS . EPOQUE ᴅᴜ ROI LOUIS XII . ᴅᴀᴘ. UN MANUSCRIT .
2. 3. SEIGNEURS VENITIENS ᴅᴀᴘ. LES FRESQUES ᴅᴇ CAMPAGNOLA, ᴀ PADOUE .
4. NICOLAS VESPUCCI CHEVALIER ᴅᴇ RHODES, ᴇᴛ ᴅᴇ LA COUR ᴅᴜ PAPE
CLEMENT VII. (1524) ᴅ'ᴀᴘ. LE BAPTEME ᴅᴇ CONSTANTIN ,
ᴀᴜ VATICAN .

PLATE 62. Beginning of 16th Century. Nobility of France and Italy. (*left*) French Gentleman of the Epoch of King Louis XII
(*middle*) Venetian Lords (*right*) Nicolas Vespucci, Knight of Rhodes, and of the Court of Pope Clement VII.

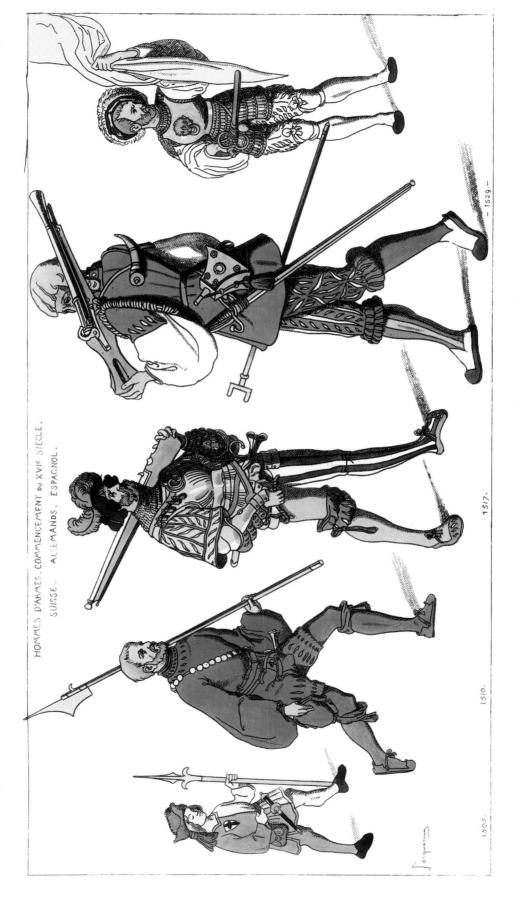

HOMMES D'ARMES. COMMENCEMENT DU XVIe SIECLE.
SUISSE. ALLEMANDS. ESPAGNOL.

PLATE 63. Men-at-Arms. Beginning of 16th Century. Swiss. German. Spanish.

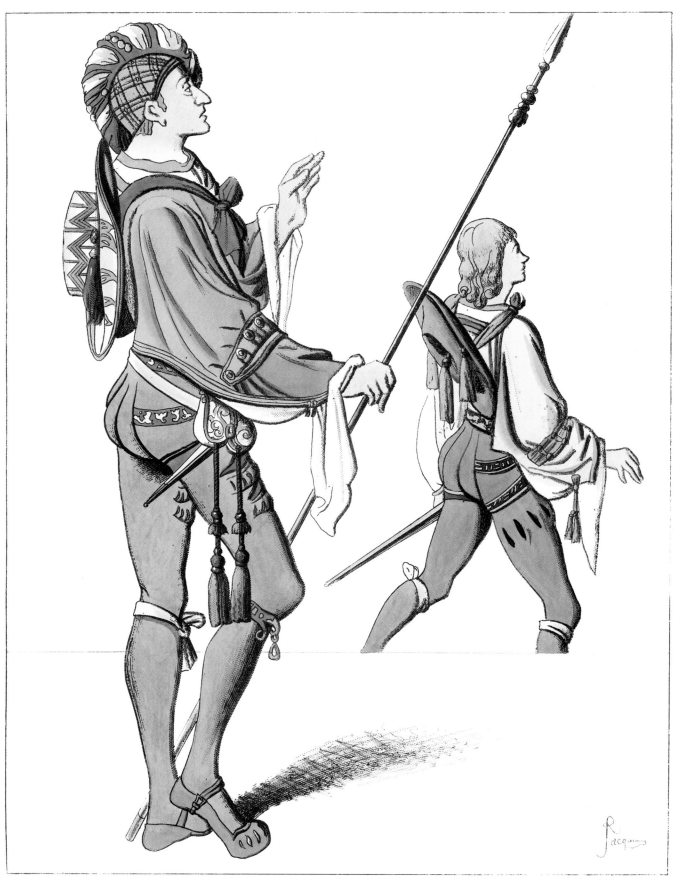

PLATE 64. Flemish Squires, 1500–15.

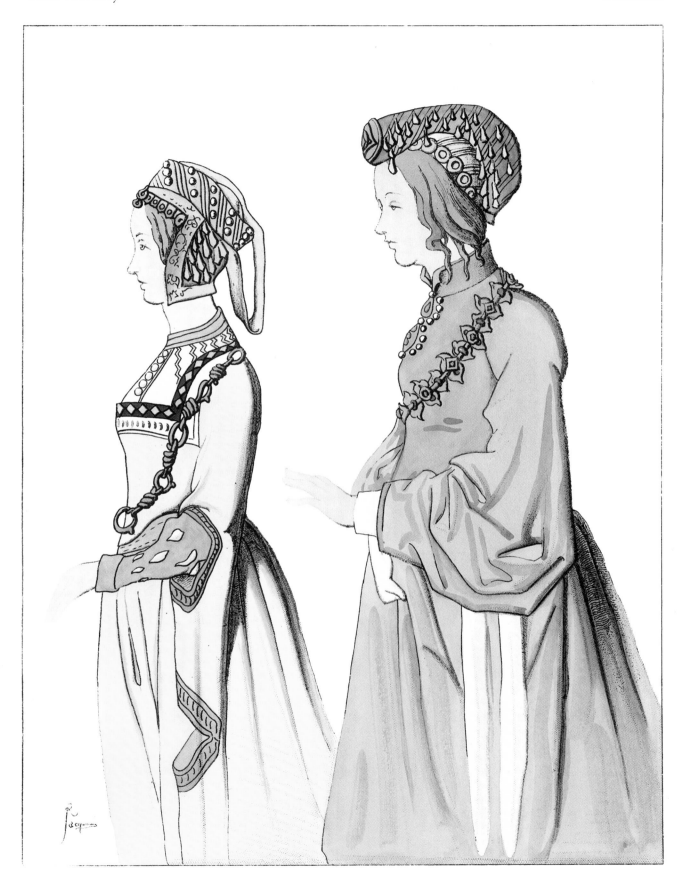

PLATE 65. Flemish Noblewomen, 1510–1520.

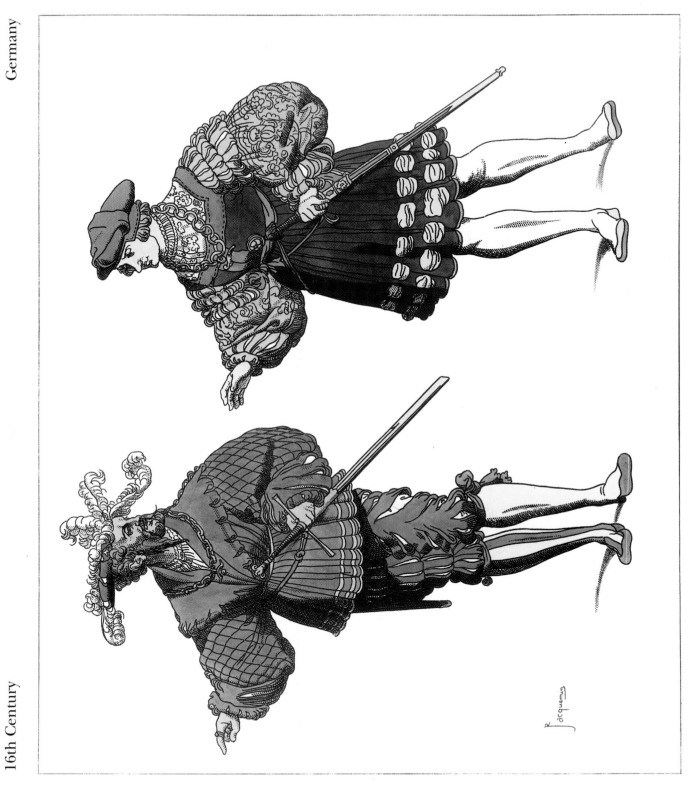

PLATE 66. German Nobility, 1515–30.

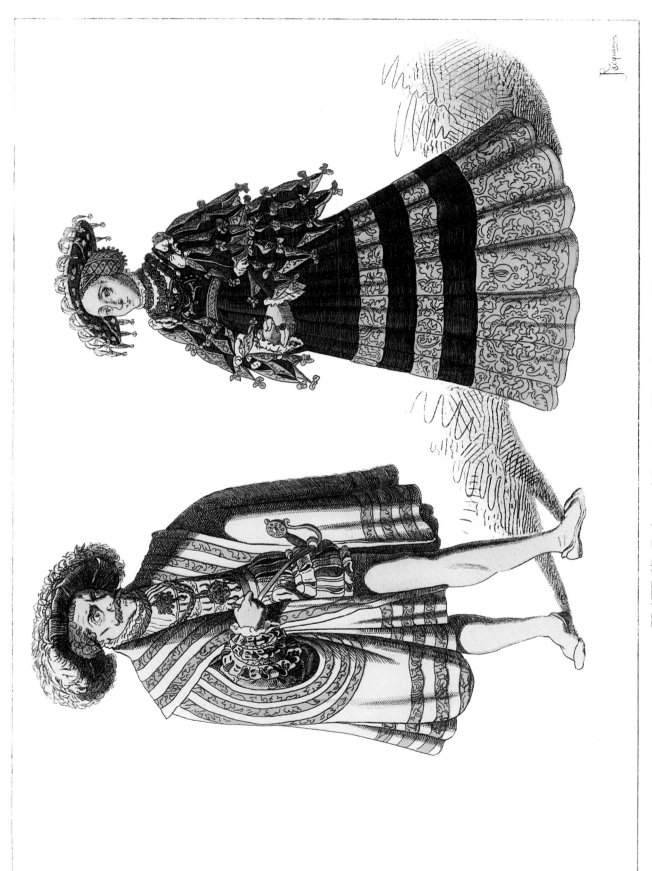

PLATE 67. Duke and Duchess of Bavaria, about 1520.

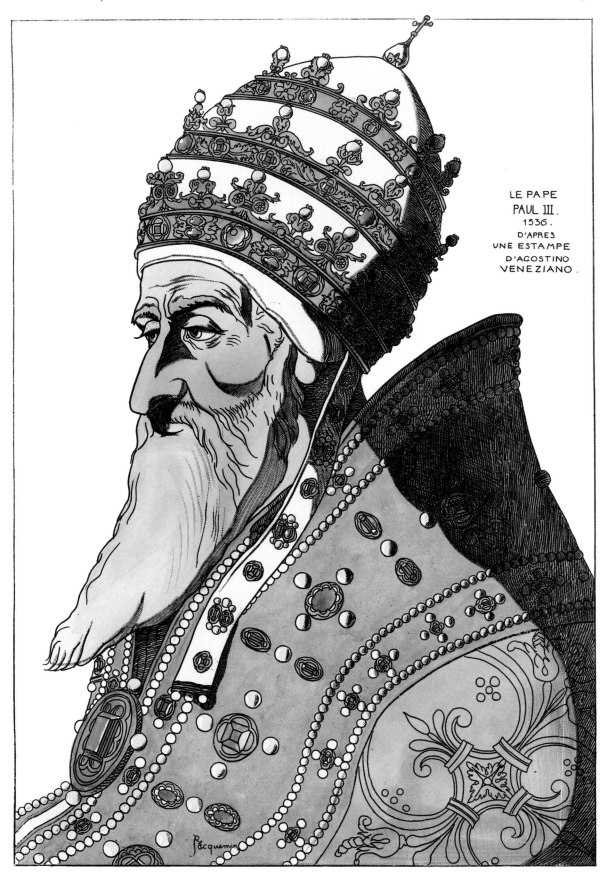

LE PAPE
PAUL III.
1536.
D'APRES
UNE ESTAMPE
D'AGOSTINO
VENEZIANO.

PLATE 68. Pope Paul III, 1536.

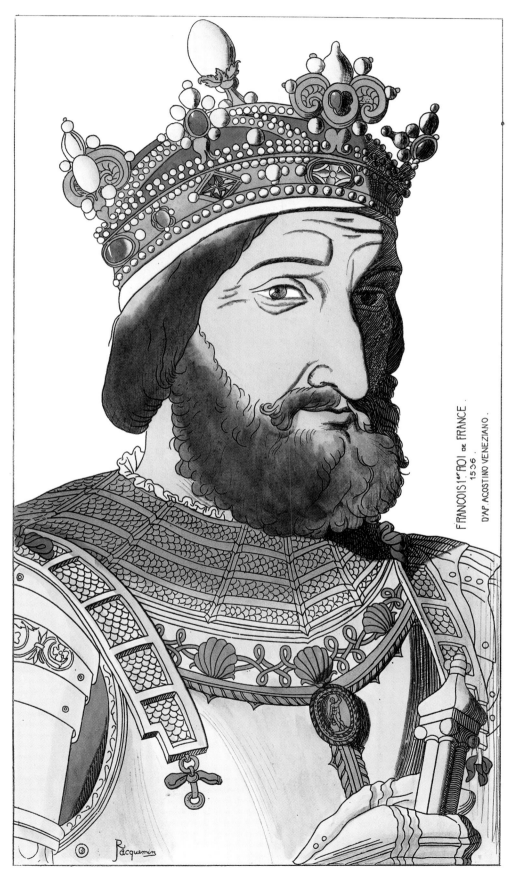

PLATE 69. François I, King of France, 1536.

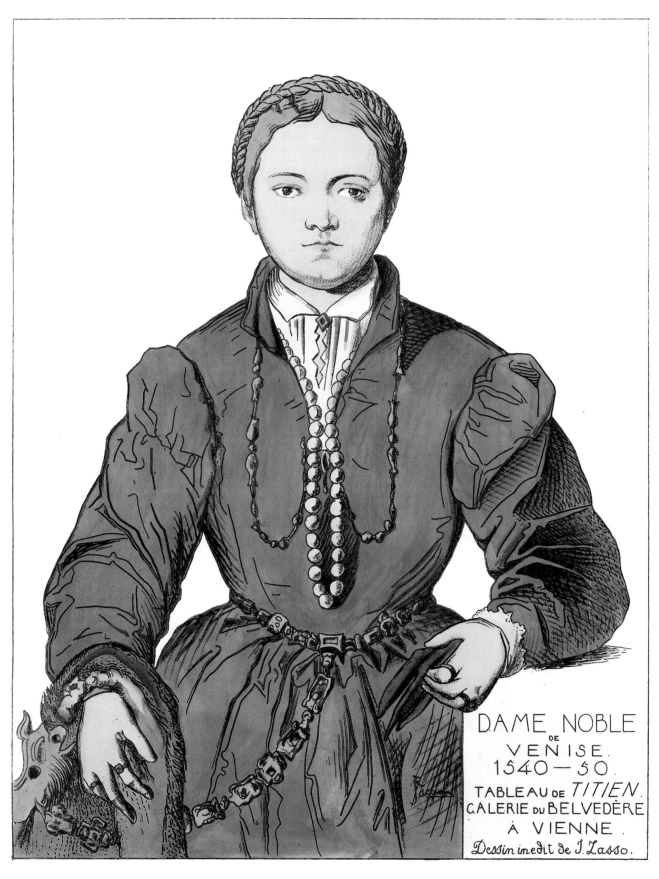

DAME NOBLE
DE
VENISE.
1540—50.
TABLEAU DE *TITIEN.*
GALERIE DU BELVEDÈRE
À VIENNE.
Dessin inedit de J. Lasso.

PLATE 70. Venetian Noblewoman, 1540–50.

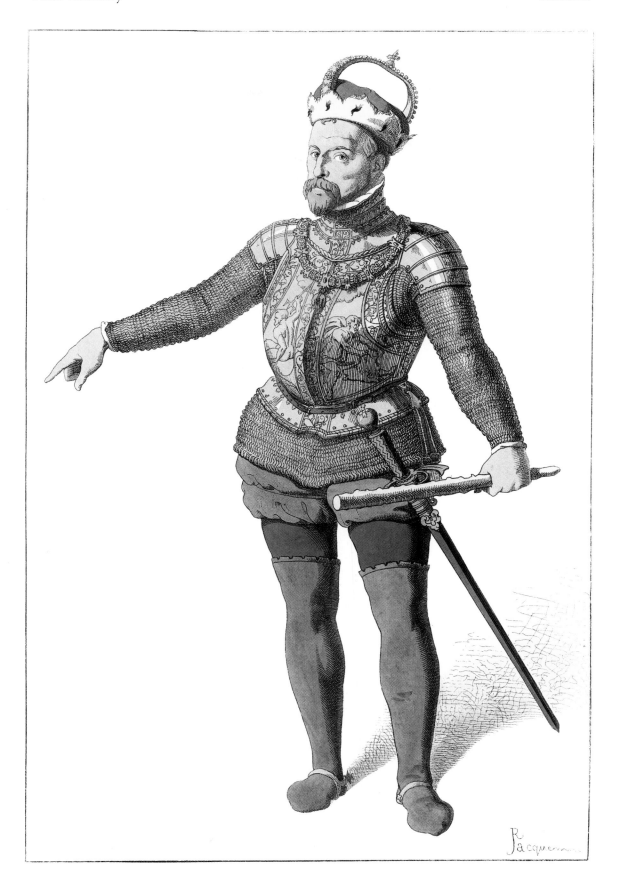

PLATE 71. Ferdinand, Archduke of Austria, Brother of Charles V.

1547.

1562.

1568.

— 1580 —

PLATE 72. French and Spanish Troops, 2nd Half of the 16th Century.

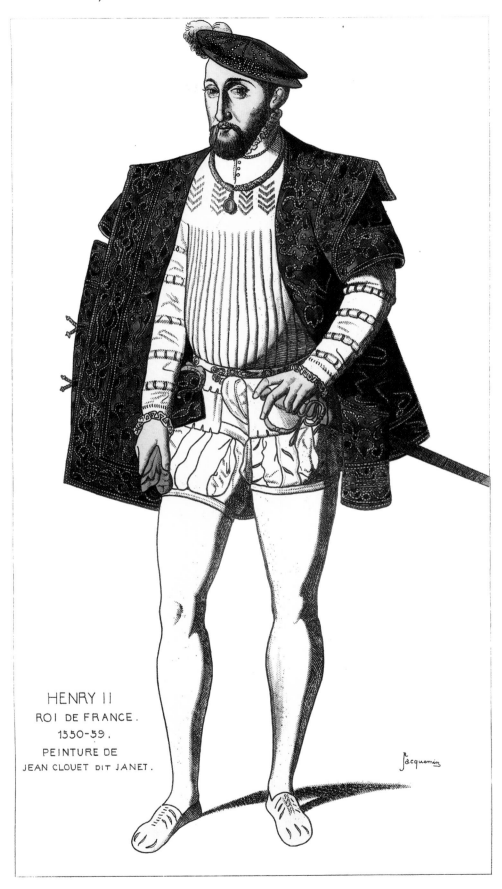

HENRY II
ROI DE FRANCE.
1550-59.
PEINTURE DE
JEAN CLOUET DIT JANET.

Jacquemin

PLATE 73. Henry II, King of France, 1550–59.

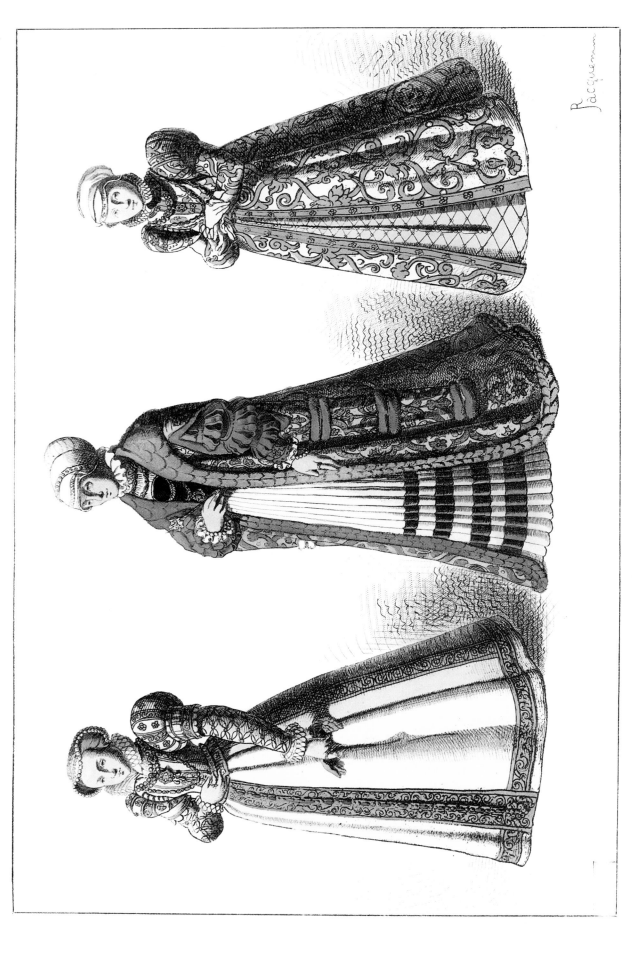

PLATE 74. Princesses of Bavaria, 16th Century.

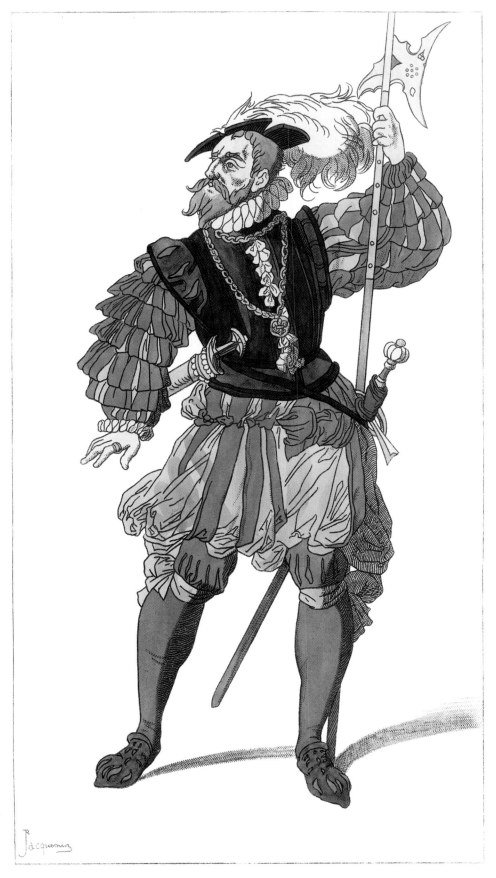

PLATE 75. Swiss Guard of the Kings of France, 2nd Half of 16th Century.

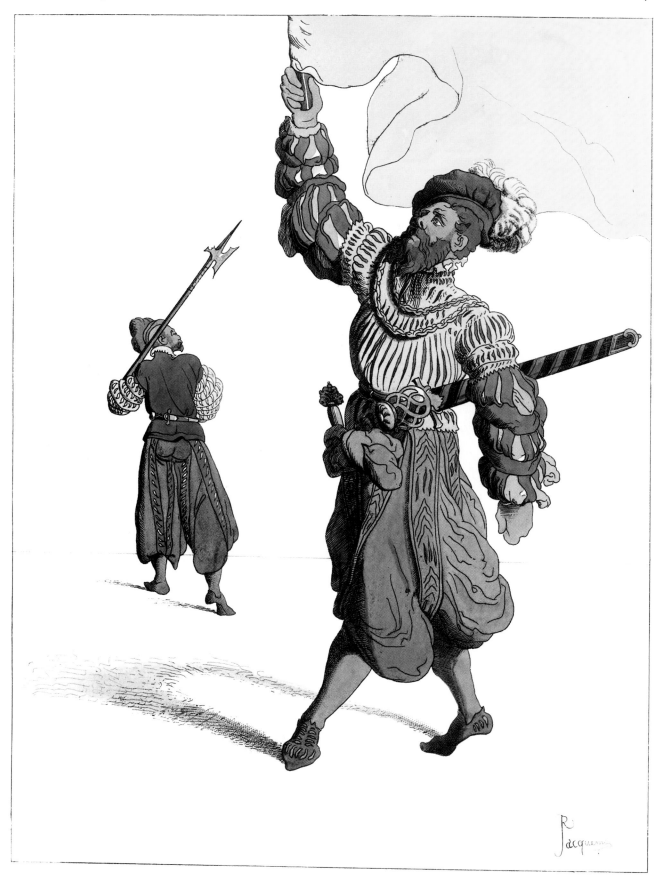

PLATE 76. German Foot Soldier, 1595. Standard-bearer.

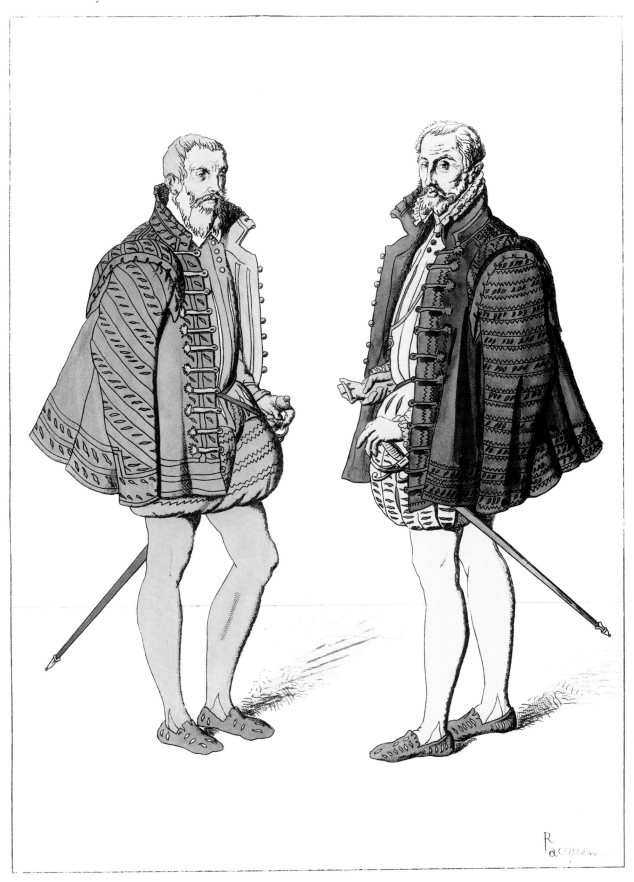

PLATE 77. Odet Cardinal de Coligny. François de Coligny.

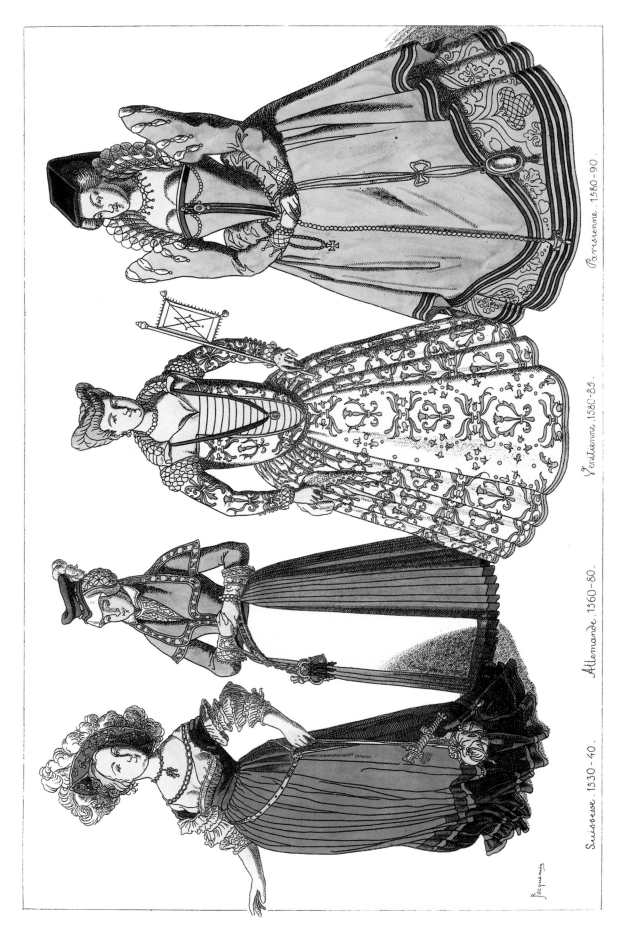

Suissesse. 1530-40.

Allemande. 1560-80.

Vénitienne. 1580-85.

Parisienne. 1580-90.

Jacquemin

PLATE 78. 16th Century. Ladies of France and Germany.

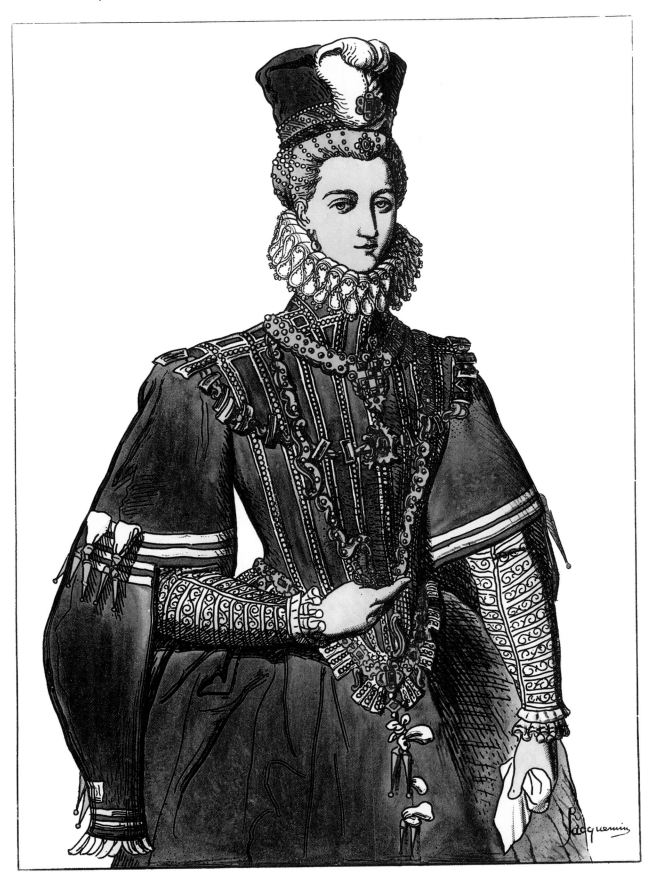

PLATE 79. Italian Princess. End of the 16th Century.

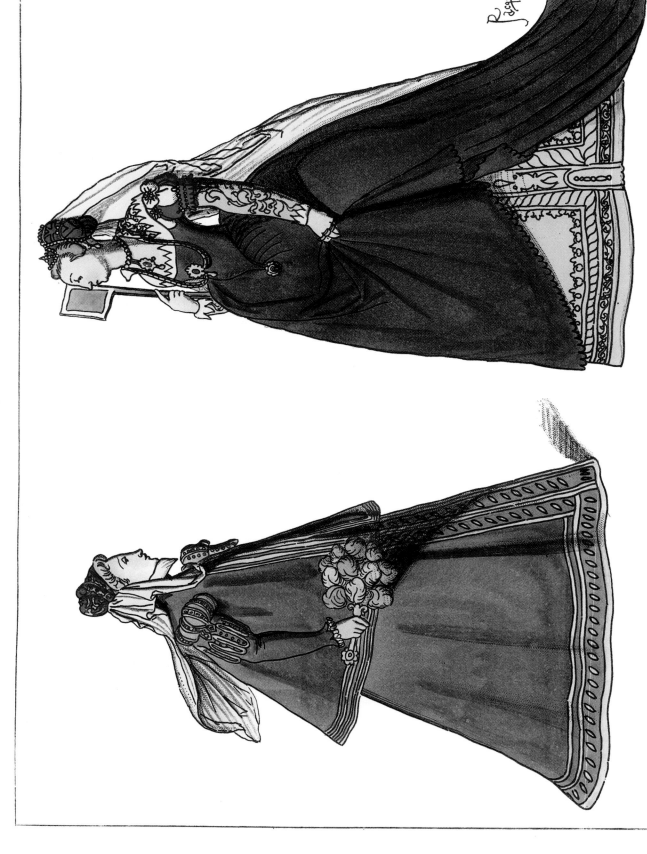

PLATE 80. Italian Ladies, 1572.

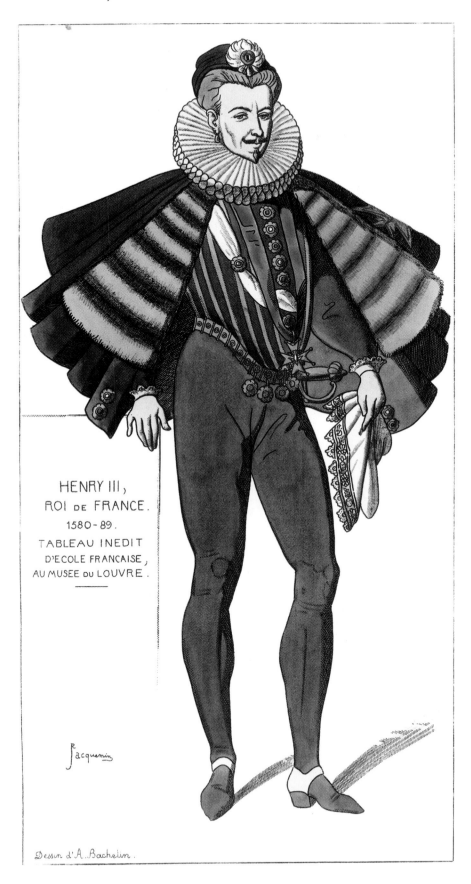

HENRY III,
ROI DE FRANCE.
1580-89.
TABLEAU INEDIT
D'ECOLE FRANCAISE,
AU MUSEE DU LOUVRE.

Jacquemin

Dessin d'A. Bachelin.

PLATE 81. Henry III, King of France, 1580–89.

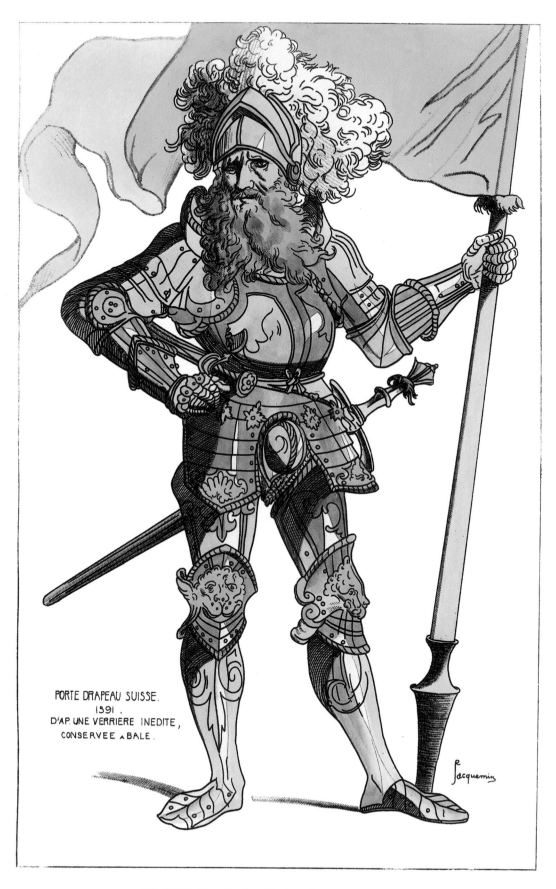

PORTE DRAPEAU SUISSE.
1591.
D'AP. UNE VERRIERE INEDITE,
CONSERVEE A BALE.

PLATE 82. Swiss Color Bearer, 1591.

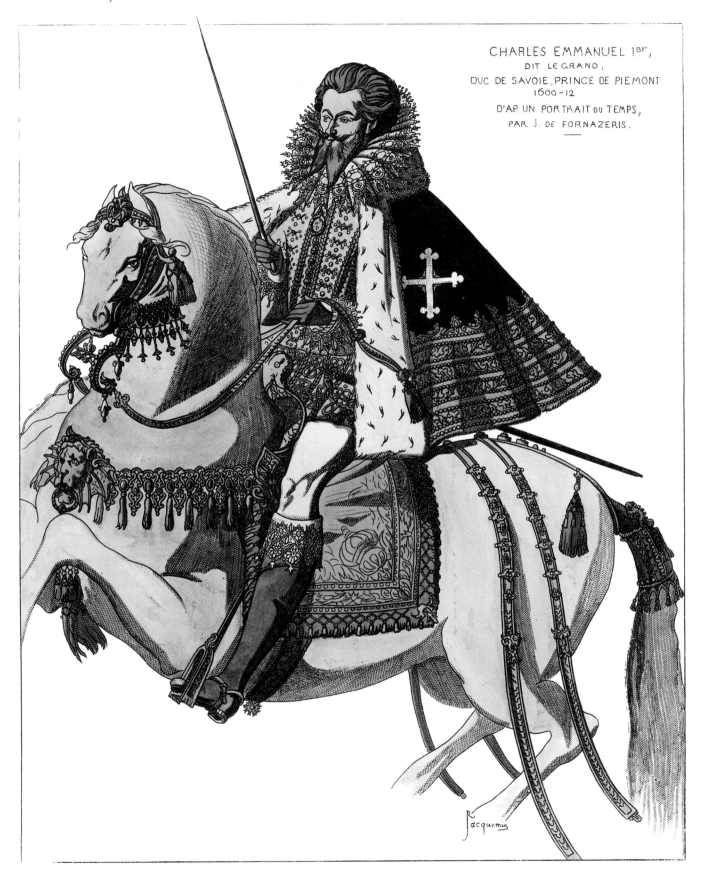

CHARLES EMMANUEL Ier,
DIT LE GRAND,
DUC DE SAVOIE, PRINCE DE PIEMONT
1600-12
D'AP. UN PORTRAIT DU TEMPS,
PAR J. DE FORNAZERIS.

PLATE 83. Charles Emmanuel I, "The Great," Duke of Savoy, Prince of Piedmont, 1600–12.

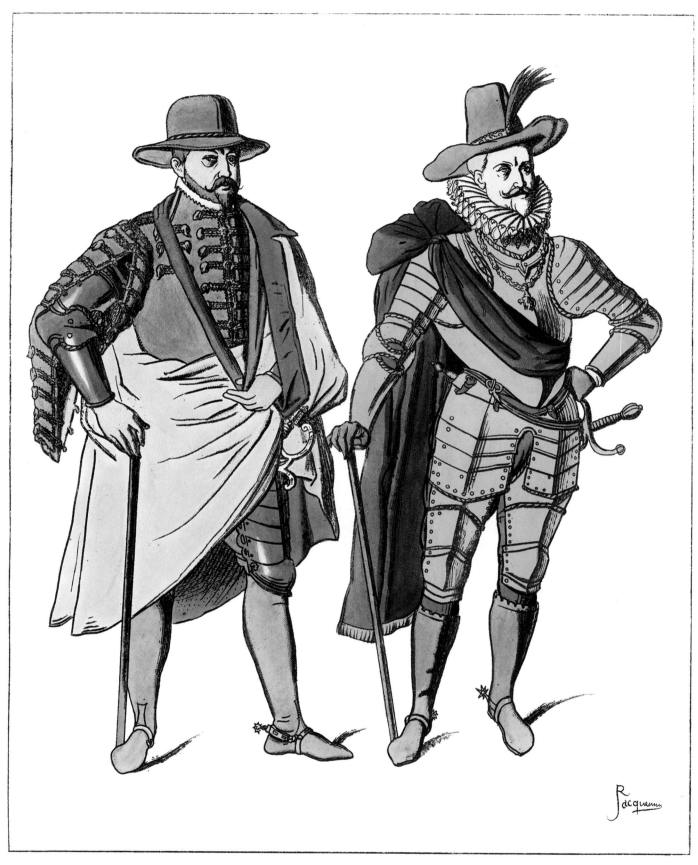

PLATE 84. André, Cardinal of Austria, Bishop of Constance (1600). Mathias,
Archduke of Austria. Duke of Wurtemburg (1601).

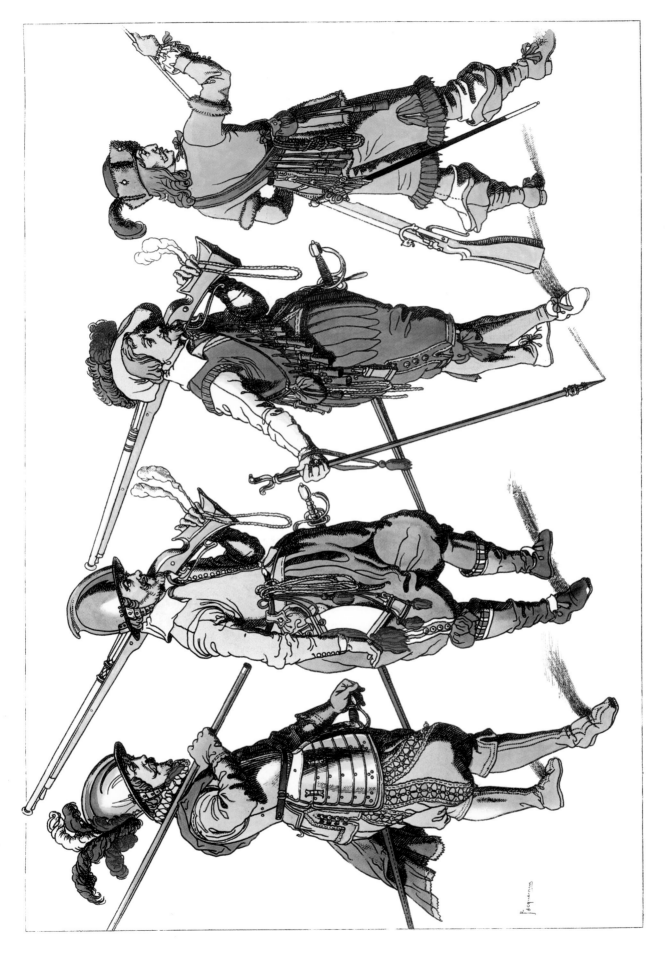

PLATE 85. Dutch Pikeman and Harquebusiers, 1608. French Musketeer, 1647.

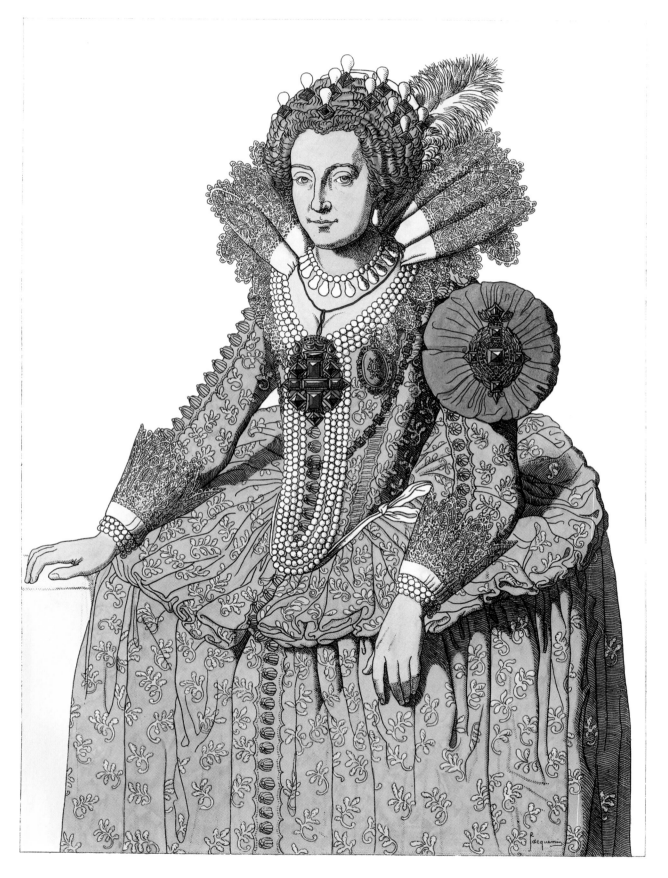

PLATE 86. Elizabeth, Palatine of the Rhine, Daughter of James I, King of England, 1612–13.

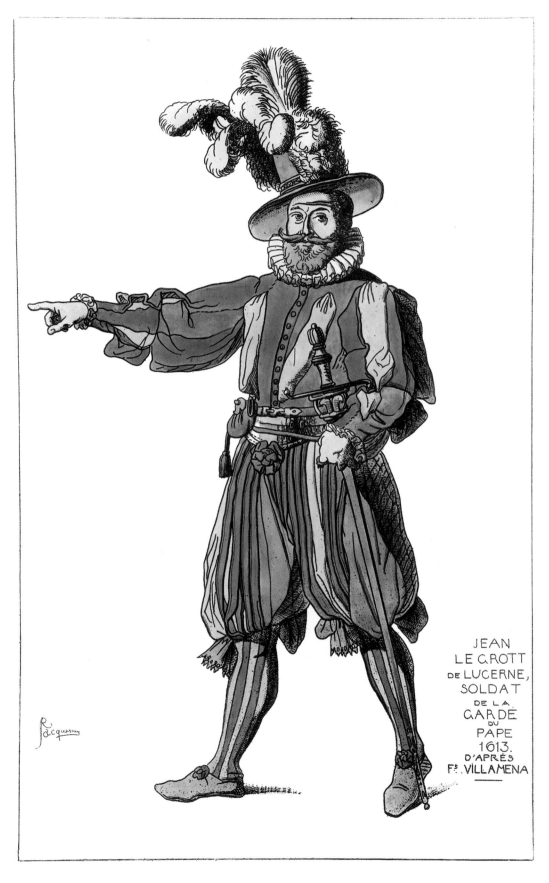

JEAN
LE GROTT
DE LUCERNE,
SOLDAT
DE LA
GARDE
DU
PAPE
1613.
D'APRÈS
Fº. VILLAMENA

PLATE 87. Jean Le Grott of Lucerne, Soldier of the Papal Guard, 1613.

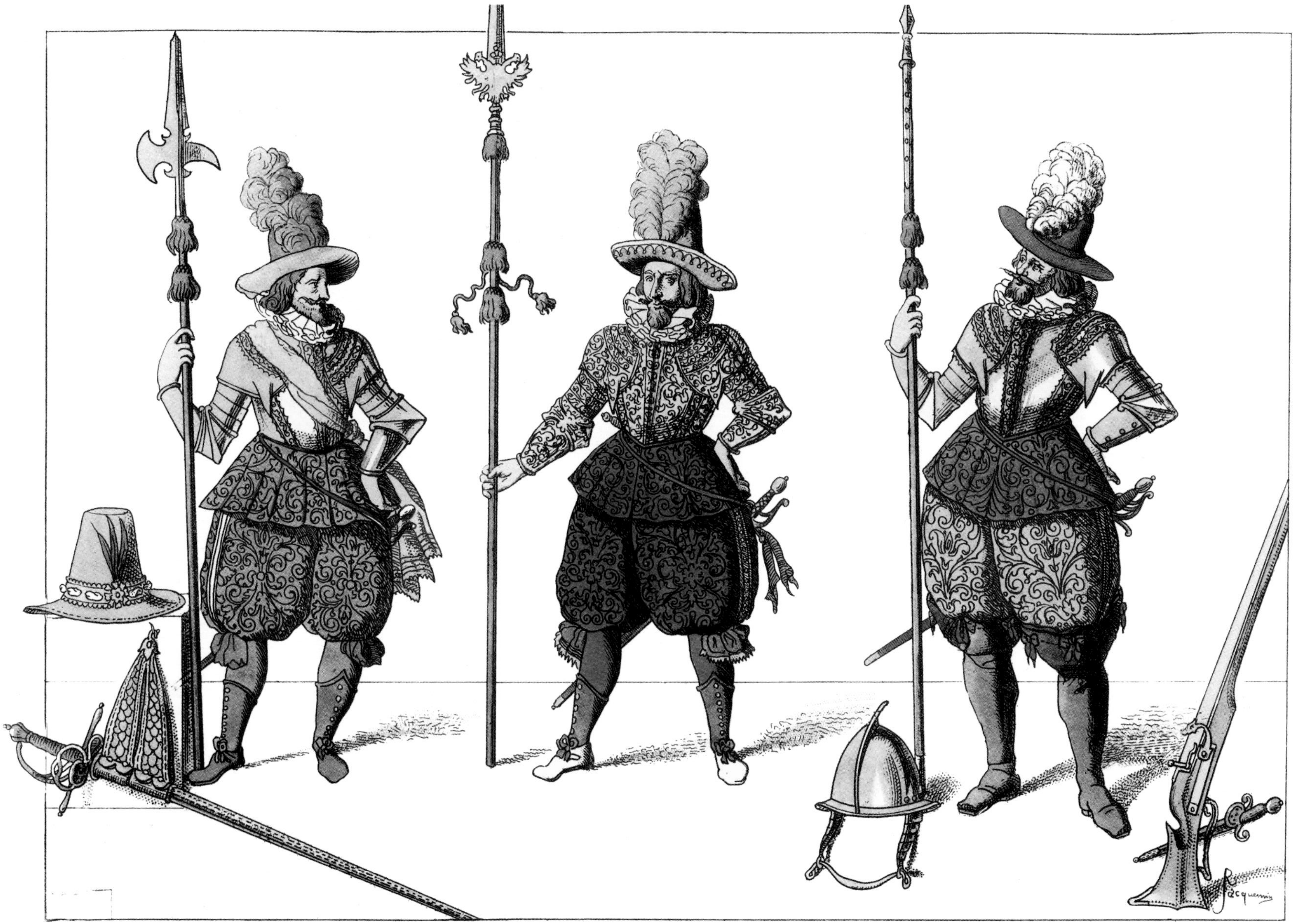

PLATE 88. Halberdiers of the Retinue of a Prince, (1615–1620).